SCREENING FOR BIOLOGICAL RESPONSE MODIFIERS:
Methods and Rationale

DEVELOPMENTS IN ONCOLOGY

F.J. Cleton and J.W.I.M. Simons, eds.: Genetic Origins of Tumour Cells. 90-247-2272-1.

J. Aisner and P. Chang, eds.: Cancer Treatment Research. 90-247-2358-2.

B.W. Ongerboer de Visser, D.A. Bosch and W.M.H. van Woerkom-Eykenboom, eds.: Neurooncology: Clinical and Experimental Aspects. 90-247-2421-X.

K. Hellmann, P. Hilgard and S. Eccles, eds.: Metastasis: Clinical and Experimental Aspects. 90-247-2424-4.

H.F. Seigler, ed.: Clinical Management of Melanoma. 90-247-2584-4.

P. Correa and W. Haenszel, eds.: Epidemiology of Cancer of the Digestive Tract. 90-247-2601-8.

L.A. Liotta and I.R. Hart, eds.: Tumour Invasion and Metastasis. 90-247-2611-5.

J. Banoczy, ed.: Oral Leukoplakia. 90-247-2655-7.

C. Tijssen, M. Halprin and L. Endtz, eds.: Familial Brain Tumours. 90-247-2691-3.

F.M. Muggia, C.W. Young and S.K. Carter, eds.: Anthracycline Antibiotics in Cancer. 90-247-2711-1.

B.W. Hancock, ed.: Assessment of Tumour Response. 90-247-2712-X.

D.E. Peterson, ed.: Oral Complications of Cancer Chemotherapy. 0-89838-563-6.

R. Mastrangelo, D.G. Poplack and R. Riccardi, eds.: Central Nervous System Leukemia. Prevention and Treatment. 0-89838-570-9.

A. Polliack ed.: Human Leukemias. Cytochemical and Ultrastructural Techniques in Diagnosis and Research. 0-89838-585-7.

W. Davis, C. Maltoni and S. Tanneberger, eds.: The Control of Tumor Growth and its Biological Bases. 0-89838-603-9.

A.P.M. Heintz, C. Th. Griffiths and J.B. Trimbos, eds.: Surgery in Gynecological Oncology. 0-89838-604-7.

M.P. Hacker, E.B. Double and I. Krakoff, eds.: Platinum Coordination Complexes in Cancer Chemotherapy. 0-89838-619-5.

M.J. van Zwieten. The Rat as Animal Model in Breast Cancer Research: A Histopathological Study of Radiation- and Hormone-Induced Rat Mammary Tumors. 0-89838-624-1.

B. Löwenberg and A. Hogenbeck, eds.: Minimal Residual Disease in Acute Leukemia. 0-89838-630-6.

I. van der Waal and G.B. Snow, eds.: Oral Oncology. 0-89838-631-4.

B.W. Hancock and A.M. Ward, eds.: Immunological Aspects of Cancer. 0-89838-664-0.

K.V. Honn and B.F. Sloane, eds.: Hemostatic Mechanisms and Metastasis. 0-89838-667-5.

K.R. Harrap, W. Davis and A.N. Calvert, eds.: Cancer Chemotherapy and Selective Drug Development. 0-89838-673-X.

V.D. Velde, J.H. Cornelis and P.H. Sugarbaker, eds.: Liver Metastasis. 0-89838-648-5.

D.J. Ruiter, K. Welvaart and S. Ferrone, eds.: Cutaneous Melanoma and Precursor Lesions. 0-89838-689-6.

S.B. Howell, ed.: Intra-Arterial and Intracavitary Cancer Chemotherapy. 0-89838-691-8.

D.L. Kisner and J.F. Smyth, eds.: Interferon Alpha-2: Pre-Clinical and Clinical Evaluation. 0-89838-701-9.

P. Furmanski, J.C. Hager and M.A. Rich, eds.: RNA Tumor Viruses, Oncogenes, Human Cancer and Aids: On the Frontiers of Understanding. 0-89838-703-5.

SCREENING FOR BIOLOGICAL RESPONSE MODIFIERS:
Methods and Rationale

James E. Talmadge, Ph.D.
NCI-Frederick Cancer Research Facility
Frederick, Maryland

Isaiah J. Fidler, D.V.M., Ph.D.
M.D. Anderson Hospital and Tumor Institute
Houston, Texas

Robert K. Oldham, M.D.
Biological Therapy Institute
Franklin, Tennessee

Martinus Nijhoff Publishing
a member of the Kluwer Academic Publishers Group
Boston/Dordrecht/Lancaster

Distributors for North America:
Kluwer Academic Publishers
190 Old Derby Street
Hingham, MA 02043

Distributors outside North America:
Kluwer Academic Publishers Group
Distribution Centre
P.O. Box 322
3300 AH Dordrecht
THE NETHERLANDS

Research sponsored by the National Cancer Institute, DHHS, under Contract No. NO1-23910 with Program Resources, Inc. The contents of this publication do not necessarily reflect the views or policies of the Department of Health and Human Services, nor does mention of trade names, commercial products, or organizations imply endorsement by the U.S. Government.

Library of Congress Cataloging in Publication Data

Talmadge, James E.

Screening for biological response modifiers.

"Research sponsored by the National Cancer Institute,
DHHS, under Contract No. NO1-23910..."—T.p. verso.
Includes bibliographies.
1. Immunotherapy. 2. Cancer—Immunological aspects.
3. Immune response—Regulation. 4. Biological
products—Testing. 5. Antineoplastic agents.
I. Fidler, Isaiah J., 1936- . II. Oldham, Robert K.
III. National Cancer Institute (U.S.) IV. Title Title: Biological response modifiers. [DNLM:
1. Adjuvants, Immunologic—therapeutic use.
2. Antineoplastic Agents—therapeutic use. 3. Drug
Screening—methods. 4. Immunotherapy. 5. Neoplasms—
therapy. QV 269 T151s]
RC271.I45T35   1985   616.99ᶜ4061   85-2990
ISBN 0-89838-712-4

Printed in the United States of America

CONTENTS

INTRODUCTION   vii

Chapter 1. Biologic and Technical Considerations for the Design
of Screening Procedures for the Assessment of
Biological Response Modifiers   1

Chapter 2. Procedures for Preclinical Screening of Biological
Response Modifying Agents   15

Chapter 3. Preclinical Evaluation of Individual Biological
Response Modifiers   121

Chapter 4. Clinical Correlations   179

v

INTRODUCTION

The observation in the 1950s that nitrogen mustard and other toxic chemicals could induce antitumor responses in patients with refractory lymphoma initiated a massive search for active chemotherapeutic agents. The initial observations stimulated a search for new chemotherapeutic agents which might have increased antitumor activity with less toxicity for normal tissues. To aid in the search for these new chemicals and to attempt to distinguish among the many toxic chemicals which might be candidates for clinical studies, the National Cancer Institute, the pharmaceutical industry, and the cancer research laboratories of most Western nations developed systems for "screening" drugs for antitumor activity. Perhaps the most extensive screening program was established by the National Cancer Institute (1). This screening program has evolved over the last two decades, an evolution which has been repeatedly reviewed (2-5). Various screening programs in use have examined over 500,000 compounds as potential anticancer agents. From these, there are now approximately forty anticancer drugs in clinical use. The utiliy of these compounds and their toxicities have been reviewed on many occasions. It is now apparent that more active and less toxic anticancer drugs are needed. It is also clear that the current screening programs are identifying compounds with similar levels of activity and with continuing moderate to severe toxicity (6).

As a result of input from a variety of sources and as a result of the recommendations of a subcommittee to the Board of Scientific Counselors of the Division of Cancer Treatment, the National Cancer Institute instituted a program to investigate biologicals and biological response modifiers in the treatment of cancer. The Biological Response Modifiers Program (BRMP) was initiated in 1980; as part of its mandate, a screening program was established to evaluate the activities and toxicities of these agents in order to form a basis for making a judgement on how to translate these agents and approaches to use in the clinic (7,8).

Like the chemotherapeutic screening program, the biological response modifier (BRM) screening program has evolved. Over the short span of its existence there have been major changes in the development of biologicals as anticancer agents. At the initiation of the program it was anticipated that interferon and perhaps one or two other recombinant biological compounds might be cloned and evaluated for clinical use within the first five years of the program. Many of the recommendations of the BRM subcommittee focused on the use of chemicals and crude extracts and the use of interferon as a natural extracted material obtained by stimulation of human white blood cells. However, the accelerating technology for the identification, cloning, and manufacturing of biological substances for use in the clinic has made available many more agents than was initially predicted by experts in the field. Therefore, there are now several families of biologicals (alpha, beta, and gamma interferon; interleukin's 1, 2, and 3; tumor necrosis factor; lymphotoxin; etc.) where one or more recombinant molecules are available. As a result, the screening process will need to establish testing programs oriented toward these compounds of biological origin in addition to small molecular weight chemicals which may influence or modulate the immune response.

Generally defined, BRM are those agents or approaches that modify the relationship between the tumor and host by modifying the host's biological response to the tumor cells with resultant therapeutic effects. BRM may modify responses in several ways:

a) Increase the host's antitumor responses through augmentation and/or restoration of effector mechanisms or mediators of the host's defense or decrease the component of the host's reaction that may be deleterious.

b) Increase the host's defenses by the administration of natural biologics (or the synthetic derivatives thereof) as effector or mediators of an antitumor response.

c) Augment the host's responses to modified tumor cells or vaccines, which might stimulate a greater response by the host or increase tumor cell sensitivity to an exisiting response.

d) Decrease the transformation and/or increase differentiation (maturation) of tumor cells.

e) Increase the ability of the host to tolerate damage by cytotoxic
modalities of cancer treatment.

Specifically BRMs include immunoaugmenting, immunomodulating, and immunorestorative agents, interferons and interferon inducers, lymphokines,
cytokines, and growth factors, thymic factors, tumor antigens, and modifiers of tumor antigen cell surface components, antitumor antibodies,
antitumor effector cells, and maturation and differentiation factors.

The Preclinical Screening Laboratory (PSL) was initiated in 1981
and has been functional for about two years. It is now appropriate to
review our rationale and comprehensive approach to the analysis of immunomodulation and therapeutic properties of BRMs. We have incorporated
an overview of data accrued from this screening program as well as
specific details of our current methodologies to provide a basis for
other program to initiate similar evaluation systems. We do not presume
that these approaches and techniques are the "best," rather they form
a functional approach to the study and comparison of immunomodulatory
and therapeutic properties of BRMs. In addition, in this monograph we
will attempt to establish preliminary data on the comparison of preclinical activity and clinical trials.

A heterogeneous mixture of chemicals, extracts, and natural and
recombinant biologicals has been tested in this screening process. A
discrete problem to be understood in this screening process has to do
with the restricted activity of certain cytokines. It is now clear
that only certain cytokines are active across species barriers. Because
of this, a screening system based in rodents will reflect biological
activity of only those cytokines which are active on rodent cells.
Since little in biology is absolute, there is also the concern that
even for those cytokines which are active in rodent systems, these
levels of activity may be very different than those seen on human
cells. Thus, there was a recommendation very early on that screening
capabilities be developed using human cells to supplement the testing
procedures being evaluated in the current screening process. While
this recommendation is sensible with respect to in vitro testing, one
is still largely restricted to animal models with respect to in vivo
activity. For those biologicals that are active only or mainly on
human cells, one can assess in vitro activity and toxicity preclin-

ically; however, the assessment of therapeutic activity requires testing in human patients. There are those biologicals which, though
inactive in rodent systems, do have some activity in subhuman primates.
This represents an additional alternative to human testing but would
be a very expensive screening system if significant numbers of biological
compounds had to be tested in primates.

This monograph will focus on the biologicals and biological response
modifiers that were available for testing between 1981 and 1984. The
compounds tested include the interferons, the thymosins, interferon
inducers, interleukin 2, bacterial extracts and products, and a variety
of small molecular weight chemicals. Monoclonal antibodies and their
immunoconjugates are a major class of biological compounds that are
being tested preclinically and translated to human trials. A systematic
screening programs for these compounds is to be initiated by the
NCI, which will include specific studies with human tumor xenografts
in nude mice, providing data on the specificity binding of monoclonal
antibody to human tumors as well as direct therapeutic activity of
immunotoxins and species specific cytokines. Since such efferts have
not been part of the PSL, no data on monoclonal antibodies will be
included in this monograph. Only preliminary clinical data are available for many of the compounds tested in the screen, which will make
correlations between the screening system and clinical activity difficult. However, for those agents and approaches which have been
tested in the clinic and for which we have some preclinical data,
correlations will be attempted. Finally, a series of conclusions
will be drawn and some recommendations regarding the screening process
will be made.

It was the initial intent of those who established the BRM screening
program to initiate a screen and test twenty to forty substances in it
to provide a data base with which to evaluate its usefulness and the
possible necessity for change. It was hoped that a substantial number
of these compounds would have been tested in the clinic so that early
correlations could also be made. At the three-year point, it is still
too early to come to definitive conclusions about the need for changes
in this screening process. At the moment, it may be best to continue
with the preclinical screen as designed and add to it from time to

time selective tests that may enlarge and expand the screening program.
Over a longer period of time, tests that appear to be less useful can
be eliminated, allowing the screening program to evolve.

The character of the BRM screening program is very different from
that of the screening program for chemotherapeutic agents. The original
design was to bring into the BRM screening program agents that had
already had some testing in other laboratories and to test them for
activity in a series of reproducible assays of increasing difficulty.
This paradigm allowed for testing of only ten to twenty agents per year
because of the scope and complexity of the testing program (9). Thus,
by design, this screening program is a focused indepth analysis of
selected BRMs as compared to the chemotherapy screening program, which
merely seeks to identify in model systems those agents which have
toxicity for selected tumor cells without undue toxicity to the host.

The need for better model systems to assess the activity of biologicals and biological response modifiers has been discussed by many
investigators (10,11). The relevance of animal models to the clinical
situation and the need for monitoring biological responses during in
vitro testing of BRMs have both been areas of some controversy with
respect to the development of this new area (12). However, there are
some studies where anticancer activity has been seen with biotherapy at
doses which were not optimal for modulating immune responses (13,14).
This raises the question of the mechanism responsible for the anticancer
activity of certain of these agents. The preclinical screen was established based on the presumption that there should be some relationship
between the biological response modifying effects of these compounds
and their clinical antitumor activity. For classical immunomodulators
this may be the case and may relate to the activity of these compounds
on only very small tumor burdens. In contrast, interferon and certain
other forms of biotherapy may have direct antiproliferative or antigrowth
activities on cancer cells and some may be directly toxic or lytic to
these cells. Such activities are more akin to chemotherapeutic agents,
but perhaps with more specificity and selectivity than has been seen
with drugs. As the clinical biotherapy data base accumulates, it may
be necessary to expand or alter the preclinical testing program to
include assays of growth inhibition and assays for cytotoxicity in the

preclinical assessment of biological materials.

In summary, the NCI's BRM Preclinical Screening Program has been active for two years. A data base has accumulated that allows one to make certain assessments of efficacy and relevance. Much of the data accumulated thus far, as summarized in this monograph, now gives the reader the opportunity to make his own assessment of this screening program. We hope that this monograph will provide information to those interested in the screening of biotherapy and immunomodulation and may prompt a reevaluation of all our screening systems so that more effective preclinical screening of anticancer agents will result. Rather than provide an extensive reference list for each BRM, we have appended to each chapter a limited number of recent reviews or comprehensive reports for each BRM.

REFERENCES

1. Goldin, A., Schepartz, S., Venditti, J. and De Vita, V. Historical development and current strategy of the National Cancer Institute Drug Development Program. Methods Cancer Res. 16:165-245, 1978.
2. Venditti, J.M. The model's dilemma. In: Design of Models for Testing Cancer Therapeutic Agents (Eds. I.J. Fidler and R.J. White), Van Nostrand Reinhold, New York, 1981, pp. 80-95.
3. Saunders, J. and Carter, S. Methods of Development of New Anti-Cancer Drugs. Natl. Cancer Inst. Monogr., 1977.
4. Goldin, A. and Venditti, J. The new NCI screen and its implications for clinical evaluation. Recent Results Cancer Res. 56:207-220, 1978.
5. Schabel, F., Griswold, D., Corbett, T., Laster, W., Mayo, J. and Lloyd, H. Testing therapeutic hypothesis in mice and man: Observations on the therapeutic activity against advanced solid tumors of mice treated with anti-cancer drugs that have demonstrated a potential clinical utility for treatment of advanced solid tumors of man. Methods Cancer Res. 17:3-51, 1979.
6. Oldham, R.K. The cure for cancer. J. Biol. Resp. Modif. 4(2), in press.
7. Oldham, R.K. Biological Response Modifiers Program. J. Biol. Resp. Modif. 1:81-100, 1982.
8. Fidler, I.J., Berendt, M. and Oldham, R.K. The rationale for and design of screening assays for the assessment of biological response modifiers for cancer treatment. J. Biol. Resp. Modif. 1:15-26, 1982.
9. Talmadge, J.E., Oldham, R.K. and Fidler, I.J. Practical considerations for the establishment of a screening procedure for the assessment of biological response modifiers. J. Biol. Resp. Modif. 3:88-109, 1984.
10. Oldham, R.K. and Smalley, R.V. Immunotherapy: The old and the new. J. Biol. Resp. Modif. 2:1-27, 1983.

11. Smalley, R.V. and Oldham, R.K. Biological response modifiers: Preclinical evaluation and clinical activity. CRC Critical Reviews in Oncology/Hematology 1:159-280, 1984.
12. Smalley, R.V. and Oldham, R.K. Interferon as a biological response modifying agent in clinical trials. J. Biol. Resp. Modif. 2:401-408, 1984.
13. Oldham, R.K. and Smalley, R.V. The role of interferon in the treatment of cancer. In: Interferon: Research, Clinical Application, and Regulatory Consideration (Eds. K.C. Zoon, P.C. Nouchi and T.Y. Liu), Elsevier Science Publishing, Amsterdam, 1984, pp. 191-205.
14. Oldham, R.K. Biologicals and biological response modifiers: Fourth modality of cancer treatment. Cancer Treat. Rep. 68:221-232, 1984.

1

BIOLOGIC AND TECHNICAL CONSIDERATIONS FOR THE DESIGN OF SCREENING
PROCEDURES FOR THE ASSESSMENT OF BIOLOGICAL RESPONSE MODIFIERS

In this chapter we present the rationale for the design of a
meaningful test system for determining the potential value of
biological response modifying agents for the treatment of cancer in
general, and metastasis in particular. For the last two centuries,
numerous efforts have focused on treating neoplastic diseases by the
manipulation of the host with agents which we now classify as
biological response modifiers (BRMs). An implicit assumption in these
studies has been the belief that clinical cancer is the consequence
of altered homeostasis, in which host responses to an oncogenic
challenge are diminished or absent. Thus, it was reasoned that the
successful awakening or boosting of a host's response to neoplasia
should lead to tumor regression. However, clinical immunotherapeutic
trials with a variety of agents have yielded discouraging results
that are greatly inferior to those obtained in various animal models.

There are several possible reasons for these poor results. In
general, animal tumor systems have relied upon the use of neoplasms
transplanted into normal syngeneic recipients. In addition, many of
these studies were actually investigating prophylaxis, since they
involved stimulation of the host before or simultaneously with tumor
implantation. Little data have been available on the ability of
syngeneic animals to reject established metastases, and even less
data are available on the outcome of immunotherapeutic studies of
metastasis in animals bearing autochthonous metastatic neoplasms.

BIOLOGIC CONSIDERATIONS

Advances in surgical and radiotherapeutic techniques and
improvements in supportive patient care have increased the success
rate for treatment of primary neoplasms, but the lethality of most
solid cancers can be attributed to their ability to produce metastases. Because metastasis has already occurred in the majority of
cancer patients at the time of diagnosis, the main problem in cancer
treatment and for BRMs is not the elimination of the primary tumor
mass, but rather the elimination or control of disseminated metas-

tases. During the process of metastasis, tumor cells come into direct contact with the various components of the immune system (natural killer cells, B cells, T cells, suppressor cells, antibodies, and macrophages). Unlike the cells within a solid tumor mass, the progenitors of metastatic foci circulate as single cells or small cell clumps and are, therefore, initially highly accessible for interaction with both immunologic and nonimmunologic host factors. Thus, on theoretical grounds, it is reasonable to predict that the immune system could be manipulated by BRMs to become highly efficient in not only inhibiting metastatic spread, but in eradicating established micrometastatic foci. In fact, BRMs may prove useful in this role without being strikingly effective against clinically apparent ("bulky") disease.

Central to the identification of BRMs useful for clinical oncology is the recognition that, in the main, the challenge is the eradication of metastases that occur in the primary host. In this regard, two important facts must be kept in mind. First, metastases do not result from the random proliferation of tumor cells shed into the circulation from the primary tumor. Rather, metastases are produced by minor subpopulations of malignant cells which preexist in the parental neoplasm. Some metastases may actually have a clonal origin, but different metastases can result from the proliferation of different progenitor metastatic cells. However, even within a metastasis of a proven clonal origin, biological heterogeneity can develop very rapidly. This, in part, may be due to the fact that highly metastatic cells exhibit an increased rate of spontaneous mutation as compared with nonmetastatic cells isolated from the same neoplasm. These data may explain the findings that cells populating a metastasis can be antigenically distinict from their parental tumor or from various other metastases. The implications of such findings as they relate to the outcome of specific immunotherapy are quite obvious. Second, normal animals are not, and should not be assumed to be, comparable to animals bearing autochthonous neoplasms. Specific or nonspecific defects may exist in animals, and correction of such defects may require a totally different form of biological modification than that required to assist the normal host in controlling neoplastic growth and metastasis.

Although the final treatment of metastasis may require the development of individualized, specific therapy, the screening of agents that modify host immunity necessitates that we first concentrate on the design of a "common-track" screen for BRMs. The term common-track denotes a standardized series of sequential assays which are relevant to many BRMs, and through which they may be screened for therapeutic potential. By no means do we suggest that all potentially effective BRMs will be identified by the use of a common-track screen. For some BRMs, such a screening procedure may be inappropriate. For the testing of those BRMs which have species specific activities, the development of suitable "specific tracks" will be required. For example, the activity of a monoclonal antibody with antitumor specificity would not be determined by using the common-track screen.

SCREENING PROCEDURE

The screening of a large number of BRM's for their therapeutic potential is an awesome task. Built into the design of our testing program is the initial capability to survey a wide range of defined biologicals and relatively pure chemical materials in a highly controlled environment. Ideally, the _in vitro_ assays employed should be predictive of the ability of a given BRM to beneficially modulate, _in vivo_, the host's innate biological responses to cancer. The recommendation that an agent be tested clinically should be based on evidence obtained from meaningful _in vitro_ and/or _in vivo_ studies that demonstrate that a BRM will aid the host in defense against cancer. The screening for BRMs may initially involve a large number of potential candidates. The screen, however, is designed to evaluate in depth a limited number of BRMs.

An ideal procedure (not presently utilized by the PSL which examines BRM's in all assays) for screening BRM for their therapeutic potential should employ a system of sequential and progressively more demanding assays designed to select a maximum number of effective agents. Those agents and less specific ones which perform well in the preliminary assays, would be tested in a more specific and discriminating manner. Once proven successful in a "second-line" assay, the agents should be tested in a third and more complex assay system, and so on. Such a step-by-step approach to the screening of potential BRM has been designed to determine their effects on T cell, B cell, NK cell, and macrophage function. The proposed sequence of progressive assays is (a) in vitro activation:in vitro testing, (b) in vivo activation:in vitro testing, and (c) in vivo activation:in vivo testing. This sequence allows the parameters of dose, schedule, route, duration and maintenance of activity, adjuvanticity, and synergistic potential to be explored in an orderly fashion for each BRM.

Initially, assays should be performed with fractionated cell populations obtained from normal donors, in order to define the baseline criteria for a positive response and to exclude the influence of tumor-induced or tumor-associated suppressor cells. The next series of assays are performed on effector cell populations isolated from animals bearing transplantable tumors with metastatic disease. Finally, because normal animals bearing transplantable tumors are not comparable to animals bearing primary tumors, another series of assays should be performed in autochthonous tumor systems, which are likely to provide the most relevant models for studies of BRM destined to be used clinically.

In Vitro Activation:In Vitro Testing.

Whether or not the results obtained from the in vitro assays are predictive for agents with in vivo antitumor activity must be determined. In vitro analysis provides only preliminary information about whether a BRM evokes a direct effect on tumor cells, or activates host immune cells to directly or indirectly affect tumor cells. Initial testing is done by adding the BRM in vitro to assess activation. Such information aids in investigating the mechanism(s) involved in eradication of neoplastic disease following treatment with the BRM.

In Vivo Activation:In Vitro Testing.

Many BRMs which interact with more than one host effector mechanism may be effective in vivo but not in vitro. For this reason it is entirely possible that the in vitro activation:in vitro testing assays may produce false negative results. The in vivo activation:in vitro testing may therefore be a more appropriate method for assessing activities of such BRMs.

In Vivo Activation:In Vivo Testing.

Initially, in vivo activation:in vivo testing procedures is used to examine the ability of BRM to enhance a host's antitumor responsiveness. Immunization is performed with nonreplicating tumor cells admixed with varying doses of augmenting agents. The efficacy of a given immunization regimen, as well as the need for multiple treatments and routes of administration, is assessed by determining the incidence of tumor growth following challenge with the specific and control tumors. Agents found to be promising in terms of their ability to increase resistance to a tumor challenge are screened further for their ability to prevent and/or eradicate experimental metastases in normal and immunosuppressed hosts. Furthermore, advantage can be taken of the recent finding that 3-week-old nude mice, whose levels of NK cell activity are low, develop metastases from injections of allogeneic and xenogeneic tumors, which include human melanoma and colon carcinoma. This predilection of the young nude mice to develop metastases can be readily reversed by a pretreatment with BRM that activate NK cells. Thus, this model can be used to assay for agents that activate and/or augment NK cells. Finally, at this level of the screening program, agents will be evaluated for their ability to eradicate spontaneous metastases produced by tumors growing in a "primary site" following implantation into syngeneic animals. Ultimately, agents found effective in these hosts are evaluated in rodents bearing autochthonous neoplasms.
Spontaneous Metastasis.

In studies investigating the therapeutic efficacy of a BRM against secondary tumor foci disseminated from a primary tumor, a reproducible and consistent secondary tumor burden needs to be obtained. This can be achieved by amputating the primary tumor and regional node(s) at a predetermined tumor volume and on the same day (also the same time following tumor initiation) for inclusion in a therapeutic cohort. To duplicate similar tumor burdens at the same time, following tumor injection, a standardized tumor cell preparation must be used. Briefly, the tumor cells must be obtained by light trypsinization from mid-log phase cultures and injected, serum-free, into healthy, age-matched, syngeneic hosts. This is in contrast to the use of tumor fragments, which can result in inconsistent tumor populations and growth rates owing to the zonal composition of tumors. The differences in the size of the tumor inoculum associated with tumor fragments can vary the induction period and growth rates, and thus prevent the use of cohorts with a consistent tumor burden.

The primary tumor needs to be inoculated at a site that can be easily resected without recurrence. This normally involves the injection of an appendage, commonly a posterior footpad or leg (muscle mass). Other sites that have been used include the ear, dermis, and subcutis. Tumors injected intradermally rapdily become necrotic owing to poor vascularity. These tumors, as well as subcutaneous tumors, may also be difficult to resect without recurrence, although this is dependent on the tumor model utilized. Because of the ease of resection, the posterior footpad is one of the most common sites of injection. In footpad injection techniques, care must be taken to prevent injection pressure from causing retrograde movement of tumor cells up the leg. The tumor-bearing leg and popliteal lymph node are amputated at a predetermined size, and the wound is drawn together using wound clips. With practice, this resection technique results in minimal mortality (<5%). Results of therapy should be reported as the percent of metastasis-negative mice and the median (range) number of metastases at a predetermined time after treatment. The long-term survival of the treated mice can also be reported.

Primary Hosts.

The importance of using primary hosts for investigating mechanisms of action of BRM that show preliminary therapeutic potential in transplantable animal tumor models cannot be overemphasized. Although this concept is generally recognized and accepted, the ability to obtain significant numbers of primary hosts in a reasonable period of time after chemical or physical carcinogenesis remains a problem. Truly spontaneous neoplasms (of unknown cause) arise in rodents, but the use of these tumors as models is currently not realistic.

The ultraviolet (UV) radiation carcinogenesis model developed by Kripke and co-workers may prove to be quite useful for studies of the effectiveness of BRM in primary hosts. In this system, chronic exposure of mice to UV radiation results in the development of single or multiple skin neoplasms. These tumors are antigenic and most are rejected when transplanted to normal syngeneic recipients. However, the tumors grow progressively in imunologically deficient recipients. In addition, UV-induced neoplasms grow progressively in syneneic mice that have been exposed to low-dose nontumorigenic UV radiation. Studies of this phenomenon revealed that the inability of UV-irradiated mice to reject challenges with syngeneic, UV-induced tumors is due at least in part, to the presence of tumor specific suppressor T cells in their lymphoid organs. The reactivity of the UV-induced suppressor cells is antigen restricted; these T cells do not suppress the rejection of either allogeneic, UV-induced tumors or even syngeneic, chemically induced tumors. Furthermore, the immune response of UV-irradiated mice to a variety of exogenous antigens is normal, suggesting that the suppressor cells show selectivity for antigens expressed on autochthonous UV-induced tumors.

The UV carcinogenesis model presents a unique system for the analysis and final testing of BRM effects on host regulatory immune mechanisms, tumor growth at a primary site, and spread to distant organs. Moreover, it is a tumor system well-suited for the testing of many agents that include immunoaugmenting, immunomodulating, and immunorestorative compounds, interferons and interferon inducers, lymphokines, cytokines, and growth factors, thymic factors, tumor antigens, and modifiers of tumor antigen cell surface components, antitumor antibodies, effector cells, and maturation and differentiation factors.

PRACTICAL CONSIDERATIONS
Positive and Negative Controls.

The need to incorporate both positive and negative controls into every assay and therapeutic study cannot be overemphasized. This will not eliminate problems, but will help detect pitfalls which can range from uniformly positive results, due for example to endotoxin contamination, to uniformly negative results related to the use of an optimized assay in which no increased activity can be induced by a BRM. Such controls will also identify intrinsic assay variation and those assays that are technical failures. A further use for positive controls is to provide a relative assessment for the quantitative ability for the test BRM to affect the assay relative to the potency of the positive control.

A positive control assumes several different forms, depending on the assay and effector cell under study. Thus, polyinosinic:polycytidylic acid (poly I:C) may provide a positive control for NK-cell and macrophage activation, but be of little use in T-cell assays. The ability of a particular BRM to stimulate a specific effector activity does not imply that it will not concomitantly stimulate other effector activities (i.e., poly I:C activates not only NK cells, but also macrophages). Therefore, assays should be designed to examine if another effector mechanism is not inadvertently being activated. A common source of error is the activity of NK cells, which can introduce spurious activity into the assays of both T-cell cytotoxicity and macrophage cytotoxicity. For these reasons, the nature, as well as the specificity, of the stimulated effector cells need to be determined, at least initially, for every assay.
Suboptimal Assay Conditions.

The investigation of a putative BRM needs to be studied within suboptimal conditions. For example, in studies dealing with the ability of a BRM to act as an adjuvant in a vaccine to prevent the growth of a tumor challenge, a highly immunogenic tumor used as a vaccine would lead to rejection of tumor challenge irrespective of any adjuvant-like activity associated with the BRM. Therefore, immunization protocols need to be suboptimal, inducing only a minimal to moderate immune response that is incapable of totally rejecting the tumor challenge unless the vaccine incorporates an effective adjuvant.

The requirement of a suboptimal assay also extends to macrophage and/or NK-cell activation. For example, virally infected mice exhibit high levels of NK-cell activity are observed. Under these conditions, the NK-cell activity may be near maximal, and a BRM is therefore unable to stimulate an increased response. We use 3-week-old mice for in vitro NK cell augmentation studies due to their low background NK activity.

Endotoxin Contamination.

One of the major problems encountered by the researcher investigating tumor immunology or tumor biology is the frequent contamination of materials and biologicals with endotoxin. Once such materials are contaminated, the biological activity of lipopolysaccharide (LPS) can sometimes be neutralized with polymyxin B, which irreversibly binds to the lipid A moiety, the biologically active portion of the LPS. However, since polymyxin B might also influence an immune assay, the best laboratory practice is undoubtedly to avoid working with reagents contaminated with LPS. Irrespective of the care one takes to prevent endotoxin contamination, it is mandatory that all materials be screened for endotoxin contamination by the Limulus lysate assay just prior to their incorporation into an assay.

STANDARDIZATION OF ASSAY CONDITIONS

Serum.

The difficulties experienced in immune assays and cell cultures which are attributed to lot-to-lot variation in serum characteristics are well documented. In addition to the utilization of a serum lot which promotes cell division and does not inhibit effector cells, consideration must be given to the type of serum used within each assay. While fetal bovine serume (FBS) or another bovine source of serum is traditionally used during in vitro assays, other serum sources, including homologous serum in rodent studies, should be considered. Studies of immune function that are dependent on the development of cytotoxic T cells may not be directed againt tumor-associated antigens (TAA), but rather against antigenic serum proteins. Homologous serum has other advantages compared with xeno-geneic serum in immune assays. The use of endotoxin-free homologous serum for supplementing medium for blastogenesis assays, mixed lymphocyte cultures, or other assays results in a low background stimulation or development of effector cells. In contrast, FBS is often blastogenic. Some of this blastogenesis has been attributed to low levels of thymosin in the serum. FBS-supplemented medium requires 5-10% serum, while studies using homologous serum must use low levels (0.5-1%) of serum supplementation owing to the toxicity of homologous murine serum.

Tumors and Tumor Cells.

Several technical considerations must be addressed when choosing a tumor model to study the activity of a BRM. Tumor lines used as stimulating and target antigens during studies of T-cell immunity can be either allogeneic or syngeneic. If a syngeneic tumor model is proposed, there is also the question of whether the tumor is of recent origin or has undergone extensive passage.

Another important consideration is the use of either a suspension cell culture or an adherent cell line. The use of an adherent tumor line requires trypsinization for harvesting and an incubation period (>4 h) to allow for the recovery of antigen expression that may have been affected by the enzymatic treatment. The kinetics of tumor cytolysis (as assayed by radioisotope release) by effector cells also differ between tumor cell lines of lymphoid origin (suspension cultures) or adherent target cell lines.

Tumor targets that are rapidly lysed, such as those of lymphoid origin (e.g. EL-4, P815,, or YAC-1), are generally assayed using a 4- to 6-hr radiorelease assay with ^{51}Cr as the radiolabel. However, the rapid spontaneous isotope release associated with adherent cell lines radiolabeled with ^{51}Cr precludes their use in the longer assays, i.e.

16 to 24 hr or longer, needed to demonstrate cytolysis. Thus we recommend that cytolysis assays with adherent targets use radioisotopes such as [^{125}I]iododeoxyuridine ([^{125}I]IUdR), [^{75}Se]methionine, [^{3}H]thymidine, ^{111}In, [^{3}H]proline, or [^{3}H]leucine. The ease of harvest and counting afforded by gamma emitters also recommends their utilization, providing that they are not radiotoxic.

The sensitivity of the proposed target to damage mediated by NK cells or macrophages must be considered in assays of specific cytotoxic T effector cells. A target line that is sensitive to NK-cell cytotoxicity may exhibit a sufficiently high background lysis to obscure specific T-cell-mediated kill. Another problem that may be avoided initially is the use of a tumor line that can produce a cytokine which could stimulate effector cell activity. An example of this problem is the production of IL-2 and other lymphokines by EL-4, or IL-1 by P388-D1.

Microbial Infections of Tumor Cells.

The use of tumor cells infected with microorganisms as target cells in immune assays or as inocula into animals has ramifications beyond in vitro cytopathogenic effects or host infection. The injection of tumor cells persistently infected with a virus or Mycoplasma may prevent tumor outgrowth due to the infection. Moreover, tumors that do develop may not metastasize at all. The rejection of virally infected cell lines is mediated by an active host process and may be abrogated by prior irradiation of the host or pretreatment of the host with anti-interferon globulin or anti-lymphocyte serum. Tumor cells infected with viruses often have increased susceptibility to killing by NK cells.

Serial Transplantation of Tumors.

The techniques used to transplant tumors are critical and influence the composition of a tumor population. Because of this, the tumor used in one laboratory may not have the same biologic characteristics as a presumably identical tumor grown in another laboratory. The mode of transplantation can also affect the cellular heterogeneity and expression of phenotypic characteristics. Most commonly, tumors are serially transplanted via trocar passage of tumor fragments. To passage a tumor, a mouse bearing the "best tumor" (e.g., a nonnecrotic tumor) is selected, and fragments from this tumor are passaged to a second group of mice. This repeated passage of tumor fragments from fast growing neoplasms may lead to the limitation or abrogation of phenotypic heterogeneity. To maintain the biological diversity of a tumor, serial transfers should be done with cell suspension obtained either by physical dissociation or preferably enzymatic digestion of tumors growing subcutaneously.

In Vitro Passage of Tumor Cells.

The in vitro passage of tumor cells can also influence its biological characteristics. No doubt, the tumor cells established in culture represent only those cells within the primary tumor that are capable of in vitro growth. This alone introduces the problem of selection. Moreover, in vitro culture of tumor cells may also modify their biological antigenic characeristics and NK susceptibility, resulting in the inadvertent selection of cellular subpopulations. For example, if a culture is harvested by trypsinization, incomplete enzymatic treatment may lead to harvesting of trypsin sensitive cells. These cells may differ in other properties from their trypsin resistant counterparts.

Environmental Conditions and Animal Care.

Lack of uniformity in animal husbandry can bring about discrepancies in experimental results. Subtle and unsuspected factors may influence the outcome of otherwise well-planned experiments. These can include hyperchlorination of drinking water or the addition of the anticaking agent silica dioxide to autoclavable feed, both of which are common husbandry techniques that depress macrophage number and function in rodents.

The macrophages of mice housed in over-crowded and dirty cages may become activated to be cytotoxic to tumor cells in vitro. Moreover, if adult male mice are removed from their cohort group and mixed with males of other groups, they fight, resulting in macrophage activation, presumably owing to the systemic induction of endotoxin following skin infection. Thus, a seemingly innocuous experimental manipulation such as mixing cohort groups of donor male mice easily influences the immune status of the test animals.

Pathogenic Viral Infections of Mice.

Rodent viruses that infect rodent colonies are ubiquitous and perturb immunological studies. Acute or early infections are immuno-stimulatory, and chronic infections are generally immunosuppressive. The viral infections demonstrated to induce immunological disturances have included most common murine viruses, notably: lactic dehydro-genase-elevating virus (LDV), lymphocytic choriomeningitis virus (LCMV), cytomegalovirus (CMV), murine hepatitis virus, and ectrome-lia. It serves little purpose to investigate the activity of a BRM in an infected animal, since data cannot be interpreted. It goes without saying that only those animals and tumors that are free of pathogenic murine viruses should be used in the screening assay for BRMs.

Histocompatibility of Recipient Animals and Tumors.

Clinical oncology concerns the pathogenesis of autochthonous tumors, which do not possess surface transplantation (histocompa-tible) antigens that differ from those of their host. Experimental studies involving transplantable (induced or spontaneous) tumors must therefore be restricted to syngeneic systems. In vivo studies of the various aspects of immune response or metastasis, which use allo-geneic systems with the concomitant strong antigenic response are probably irrelevant.

CONCLUSIONS

A successful BRM screen should identify those agents useful for treatment of human cancer. The preclinical screen for BRM must provide an understanding of their mechanism and optimal scheduling in addition to the mere demonstration of effectiveness. The preclinical screen for BRM that we have developed can be viewed as a continuum, beginning with in vitro assays of immunomodulation and progressing to studies of in vivo stimulation assayed in vitro and then on to the investigation of immunotherapeutic potential. These immunotherapy models also represent a continuum from the straightforward and convenient transplantable tumor models to a more stringent test of BRM function, the development of an objective response against primary, carcinogen-induced autochthonous tumors. We anticipate that the testing of BRM in an evolving, controlled system will ultimately contribute to the development of novel approaches for the treatment of clinical cancer.

Note: For detailed information regarding particular subjects discussed in this chapter, the reader is referred to our previous publications:

Fidler, I.J., Berendt, M., Oldham, R.K. The rationale for and design of a screening procedure for the assessment of biological response modifiers for cancer treatment. J. Biol. Resp. Modif. 1982, 1:15-26.

Talmadge, J.E., Oldham, R.K., and Fidler, I.J. Practical considerations for the establishment of a screening procedure for the assessment of biological response modifiers. J. Biol. Resp. Modif. 1984, 3:88-109.

2

PROCEDURES FOR PRECLINICAL SCREENING
OF BIOLOGICAL RESPONSE MODIFYING AGENTS

Table of Contents

Page #

	TABLE OF CONTENTS	15-22
	GLOSSARY	23-24
1.000	ANIMALS AND ANIMAL CARE	25
1.100	Supplier	25
1.200	Animals	25
1.300	Housing	25
1.400	Control	25
1.500	Age	25-26
2.000	TUMOR CHARACTERISTICS	26
3.000	IN VIVO TECHNIQUES	26
3.100	Intravenous Injection	26
3.101	Standardization of Cell Suspension	26-27
3.102	Intravenous Injection of Tumor Cells	27-28
3.103	Enumeration of Pulmonary Colonies	28
3.200	Footpad Injection	28-29
3.201	Amputation	29
3.202	Footpad Measurement	29
3.300	Intraperitoneal Injection	29
3.400	Subcutaneous Inoculation	29-30
3.401	Monitoring of Subcutaneous Tumors	30
3.500	Intradermal Injection	30
3.600	Filling the Syringe	30-31
3.700	Necropsy	31-32
3.800	Thymectomy	32
3.801	Adolescent Mice	32
3.801a	Reagents	32
3.801b	Materials	32
3.801c	Procedure	33-34
3.802	Neonatal Mice	34

15

3.802a	Materials	34
3.802b	Procedure	35
3.900	Bleeding of Mice	35
3.901	Tail Bleeding	35
3.902	Cardiac Puncture	35-36
3.903	Subaxillary Bleeding	36
3.904	Puncture of the Retro - Orbital Plexus	36-37
4.000	TISSUE CULTURE PROTOCOLS	37
4.100	Reagents	37
4.200	Preparation of Tissue Culture Medium	38
4.201	Complete Minimum Essential Medium (CMEM)	38
4.202	Complete EMEM (methionine free)	38
4.203	Complete Williams medium E	38
4.204	Complete RPMI-1640	38
4.205	Extra high amino acids (EHAA) medium	38-39
4.205a	Stock nucleic acid precursors (100X)	39
4.205b	Preparation of normal mouse serum (NMS)	39
4.206	Medium for P815	39
4.300	Cell Cryopreservation Medium	40
4.400	Preparation of Assay Reagents	40
4.401	[^{125}I]IUdR	40
4.402	[^{3}H]Proline	40
4.403	[^{75}Se]Methionine	40
4.404	[^{3}H]Thymidine	40
4.405	1% Triton X-100	40
4.406	2% Sodium Dodecyl Sulfate (SDS)	40
4.407	0.1 M Sodium Hydroxide (NaOH)	40
4.408	White Blood Cell Counting Fluid (WBCF)	40
4.409	Trypan Blue Stain (0.4%)	41
4.410	Mitomycin C	41
4.411	2-Mercaptoethanol (2-ME)	41
4.412	Trypsin-EDTA Solution	41
4.413	Phosphate Buffered Saline-Tween (PBS-Tween)	41
4.414	Carbonate Coating Buffer	41
4.415	10% Diethonolamine Buffer	42

4.416	Substrate Solution	42
4.500	Harvesting of Adherent Tumor Cells	42
4.600	Radiolabeling of Tumor Cells	43
4.601	[^{125}I]IUdR Labeling	43
4.602	[^{3}H]Proline Labeling	43-44
4.603	^{51}Cr Labeling	44
4.604	^{111}In Labeling	44-45
4.700	Cryopreservation of Cells	45-46
4.800	Mitomycin C Treatment of Cells	46
4.900	Heat Inactivation of FBS	46
4.1000	Establishment of Primary Cultures	46-47
4.1100	General Cytotoxicity Assay	47
4.1200	Growth Curves	48
5.000	QUALITY CONTROL	48
5.100	Testing of Media	48-49
5.200	Testing of Sera	49
5.300	Testing for the Presence of Endotoxin	49
5.301	Reagents and Materials	49
5.302	Procedure	50
5.400	Contamination of Cell Lines	50
5.500	Testing of [^{125}I]IUdR Stock	50-51
6.000	CELLULAR PREPARATIONS EX VIVO	51
6.100	Preparation of Lymphoid Cell Suspensions	51
6.101	Reagents	51
6.102	Materials	51-52
6.103	Procedure	52-53
6.200	Collection of Mouse Peritoneal Macrophages (Resident Macrophages)	53
6.201	Reagents	53
6.202	Materials	53
6.203	Procedure	54-55
6.300	Collection of Mouse Peritoneal Exudate Cells (Thioglycolate Elicited)	55
6.400	Collection of Rat Alveolar Macrophages	55
6.401	Reagents	55

6.402	Materials	55
6.403	Procedure	56-58
6.500	Collection of Mouse Alveolar Macrophages	58
6.501	Materials	58-59
6.502	Preparation for Lavage	59-60
6.503	Lavage	60
6.600	Collagenase Dissociation of Tumors	61
6.601	Reagents	61
6.602	Materials	61
6.603	Tumor Excision	61-62
6.604	Dissociation	62
6.700	Cryopreservation of Collagenase-Dissociated Cell Suspensions	62
6.701	Cell Preparation	62-63
6.800	X-Irradiation of Tumors Cells	63
6.801	Preparation of Cells	63
6.900	Cloning by Limiting Dilution in Micro Test II Plates	63-64
6.1000	Preparation of Mononuclear Cells from Blood or the Separation of Viable Cells from a Mixed Cell Population	64
6.1001	Reagents and Equipment	64
6.1002	Procedure	64-65
6.1100	Murine Peripherial Blood Lymphocyte	65
6.1200	Isolation of Pulmonary NK Cells	65
6.1201	Equipment	65-66
6.1203	Procedure	66
6.1300	Isolation of Hepatic NK Cells and Kupffer Cells	66
6.1301	Equipment	66-67
6.1302	Reagents	67
6.1303	Procedure	67
6.1400	Isolation of Large Granular Lymphocytes by Percoll Density Gradient Centrifugation	67
6.1401	Reagents	68
6.1402	Equipment	68
6.1403	Procedure	68
7.000	TECHNIQUES USED IN MECHANISM STUDIES	68
7.100	Preparation and Use of Nylon Wool Columns for T-Cell Enrichment	68
7.101	Reagents	68

19

7.102	Materials	68-69
7.103	Procedure	69
7.103a	Washing and Drying of Nylon Wool	69
7.103b	Packing of Nylon Wool Columns	69-70
7.103c	Cell Separation	70-71
7.200	Preparation of Liposomes: Multilamillar Vesicles (MLV)	72
7.201	Equipment	72
7.202	Reagents	72
7.203	Preparatory Steps	72
7.203a	Washing of Glassware	72
7.203b	Preparation of Lipid	72-74
7.204	Preparation of Liposomes	74-75
7.500	Determination of Cl Content	75
7.501	Reagents and Materials	75
7.502	Assay of Cl Content	75
8.000	ALLOGENEIC MIXED LYMPHOCYTE REACTION (MLR) ASSAY	75
8.100	Reagents	75
8.200	Materials	76
8.300	Procedure	76
8.400	Plating	76-77
8.500	Representation of Data	77-78
9.000	ALLOGENEIC MIXED LYMPHOCYTE TUMOR REACTION - CELL-MEDIATED CYTOTOXICITY (MLTR - CMC)	78
9.100	Reagents	78
9.200	Materials	78
9.300	Treatment of P815 Cells	78
9.400	Preparation of MLTR-CMC Spleen Cells	79
9.500	Incubation of MLTR-CMC	79-80
9.600	Cytotoxicity Testing of MLTR-CMC (4-hr ^{51}Cr-Release Assay)	80
9.601	^{51}Cr-Labeling of P815 Target Cells	80
9.602	Plating of MLTR-CMC 4-hr ^{51}Cr-Release Assay	80-81
9.700	Calculation of Percent Cytotoxicity	81
10.000	SUPPRESSOR CELL-HELPER ASSAYS	81
10.100	Reagents	81
10.200	Materials	81-82
10.300	Incubation of a Second MLTR Culture	82
11.000	MEMBRANE PHENOTYPE OF REGULATORY OR EFFECTOR CELLS	82
11.100	Reagents	82-83

11.200	Materials	83
11.300	Antibody Treatment	83
12.000	CELL-MEDIATED CYTOTOXICITY ASSAY (CTL)	84
12.100	Reagents	84
12.200	Materials	84
12.300	Immunization	84-85
12.400	Preparation of Target Cells	85
12.500	Assay	86
13.000	NK CELL ASSAY	86
13.100	In Vitro Incubation of Spleen Cells with NK Activation	86
13.101	Reagents	86
13.102	Materials	87
13.103	Preparation of Spleen Cells	87
13.104	Incubation of Spleen Cells with Potential NK Activators	87-88
13.200	NK Cell Assay: ^{51}Cr Release	88
13.201	Reagents	88
13.202	Materials	88
13.203	^{51}Cr Labeling of YAC Target Cells	88
13.300	Preparation of In Vivo Activated NK Cell	88-89
13.301	Short-Term - ^{51}Cr-Release Assay	89-90
13.302	Calculation of Percent Cytotoxicity	90
13.400	NK Cell Assay: Long-Term - [^{3}H]Proline	90
13.401	Reagents	90
13.402	Materials	90
13.403	[^{3}H]Proline Labeling of UV-2237 Target Cells	91
13.404	Preparation of NK Spleen Cells	91
13.405	Plating of Long-Term [^{3}H]Proline Assay	91-92
13.406	Calculation of Percent Cytotoxicity	92
13.500	Determination of the Kinetics of NK Cell Activation and the Potential to Sustain NK Cell Activity	92
13.501	Kinetics	92
13.502	Sustaining Activity	92-93
14.000	MACROPHAGE MICROCYTOTOXICITY ASSAYS	93
14.100	Reagents	93
14.200	Materials	93

14.300	Plating of 72-hr Macrophage Microcytotoxicity Assay	93-95
14.400	Harvesting of 72-hr Microcytotoxicity Assay	95
14.500	Calculation of Percent Cytotoxicity (Using Mean Value of Triplicates)	95
14.600	^{111}In Labeling of Target Cells	95
14.700	Plating of ^{111}In Release Macrophage Microcytotoxicity Assay	95-97
14.800	Harvesting of ^{111}In Release Microcytotoxicity Assay	97
14.900	Calculation of Percent Cytotoxicity (Using Mean Value of Triplicates	97
15.000	B-CELL ASSAYS	97
15.100	Hemagglutination Assay	97
15.101	Reagents	97
15.102	Materials	97
15.103	Procedure	97-98
15.200	Murine Lymphocyte Proliferation Assay	98
15.201	Reagents	98
15.202	Materials	98
15.203	Procedure	98-99
15.300	Adjuvant Activity for B Cells (Enzyme-Linked Immunosorbent, Assay)	99
15.301	Reagents	99
15.302	Materials	99-100
15.303	Immunization and Serum Collection	100
15.304	ELISA assay	100-101
16.000	BRIEF REVIEWS OF IMMUNOMODULATORY PROTOCOLS	101
16.100	T-Lymphocyte Assays	101-102
16.101	In Vitro Activation: In Vitro Testing	102-103
16.102	In Vivo Activation: In Vitro Testing	103
16.200	B-Cell Assays	103-104
16.201	In Vitro Activation: In Vitro Testing	104
16.202	In Vivo Activation: In Vitro Testing	104
16.300	Natural Killer (NK) Cell Assays	104
16.301	In Vitro Activation: In Vitro Testing	104
16.302	In Vivo Activation: In Vitro Testing	104-105
16.400	Macrophage Assays	105
16.401	In Vitro Activation: In Vitro Testing	105

22

16.402	In Vivo Activation: In Vitro Testing	105-106
17.000	THERAPY MODELS OF TRANSPLANTABLE TUMORS	106-107
17.100	Adjuvant Activity of the BRM: Induction of a Specific Cytotoxic T-Cell Response	107
17.200	Ability of a BRM to Stimulate Effector T-Cell Activation in the Presence of Suppressor T Cells	107
17.300	Ability of a BRM to Activate Nonspecific Effector NK Cells In Vivo and Decrease the Formation of Pulmonary Tumor Nodules	108
17.400	Therapy of Established Metastases	108-109
17.401	Testing Protocol	109
18.000	TESTING OF BRM IN AUTOCHTHONOUS TUMOR MODELS	109
18.100	UV Carcinogenesis	109-111
18.200	NMU Carcinogenesis	111-112
19.000	POSITIVE CONTROLS	113
19.100	T-Cell Assays	113
19.200	NK Cell Assays	113
19.300	Macrophage Assays	113
19.400	B Cell Assays	113
19.500	Therapy	113
	APPENDIX	114-117
	REFERENCES	118-119

GLOSSARY

AM - alveolar macrophage

BRM - biological response modifier(s)

CMEM - complete minimum essential medium (Eagle's)

CMF-HBSS - Ca^{++}- Mg^{++}-free Hanks' balanced salt solution

cpm - counts per minute

CTL - cytotoxic T lymphocytes

DMSO - dimethylsulfoxide

EAA - essential amino acids

EHAA - extra high amino acids

EMEM - Eagle's minimum essential medium

FBS - fetal bovine serum

ΔFBS - heat-inactivated fetal bovine serum

HBSS - Hanks' balanced salt solution

HEPES - HEPES buffer

i.d. - intradermal

i.p. - intraperitoneal

i.v. - intravenous

$[^{125}I]$IUdR - $[^{125}I]$iododeoxyuridine

LPS - lipopolysaccharide

MDP - muramyl dipeptide

2-ME - 2-mercaptoethanol

MEM - minimum essential medium (Eagle's)

MLR - mixed lymphocyte reaction

MLTR - mixed lymphocyte tumor reaction

MLV - multilamillar vesicle(s)

MΦ - macrophage

MTP-PE - muramyl tripeptide-phosphatidylethanolamine

NEAA - nonessential amino acids

NK - natural killer

NMU - N-methyl-N-nitrosourea

PC - phosphatidylcholine

PCS - phase combining scintillation fluid

PEM - peritoneal exudate macrophages

23

PFC - plaque-forming cells

Poly I:C - polyinosinic:polycytidylic acid

PM - peritoneal macrophage

PS - phosphatidylserine

PWM - pokeweed mitogen

RPI - relative proliferation index

RPM - revolutions per minute

RPMI - Roswell Park Memorial Institute - 1640 medium

s.c. - subcutaneous

SI - stimulation index

SDS - sodium dodecyl sulfate

SPC - spleen cells

SRBC - sheep red blood cells

UV - ultraviolet light

WBC - white blood cell

WBCF - white blood cell counting fluid

1.000 ANIMALS AND ANIMAL CARE

1.100 Supplier
Purchase animals from a supplier guaranteeing them to be specific
pathogen free.

1.200 Animals
BALB/CanN mice
BALB/CanN-nu mice
C3H/HeN (MTV-) mice
C57BL/6N mice
DBA/2
F344 rat
Sprague Dawley rat (CAMM)

1.300 Housing
There should be three classes of containment for the animals:
(1) a holding barrier for nonexperimental animals, access to which
is limited to authorized personnel, (2) an experimental barrier
that contains quarantine rooms, access to which is limited to
authorized personnel wearing protective clothing, and (3) conven-
tional housing for most of the experimental animals, allowing
free access but maintaining a SPF- and virus-free colony.

1.400 Controlled Environment
All experimental animals should be given identical environmental
conditions and care. Lack of uniform housing, diet, etc. can be
the source of discrepancies in experimental results, e.g., a crowded
and/or a dirty environment can stimulate both NK-cell cytotoxicity
and macrophage cytotoxicity. Thus, for certain critical experiments,
mice should be obtained the same day of weaning and kept in uncrowded
conditions. Furthermore, because of the immunosuppressive and/or
immunostimulatory nature of viral infections, all mice should be
obtained and maintained free of known pathogenic viruses.

1.500 Age
The mice within each experiment must be matched for age and sex. Mice
used in NK-cell assays or therapy should be freshly weaned and used at
21 days of age. Routinely, mice should be obtained at 4 wk of age and

used between 6 and 8 wk of age for tumor therapy studies. Donor mice for AM studies should be 12-14 wk old.

2.000 TUMOR CHARACTERISTICS

Tumor Lines

Tumor	Classification	Origin	Induction Agent
A375 (1)	melanoma	human	unknown
K562 (2)	leukemia	human	unknown
MADB-200 (3)	mammary adenocarcinoma	F344 rat	9,10-dimethyl-1,2 benzanthracene
B16-BL6 (4)	B16 melanoma variant	C57BL/6 mouse	unknown
P815 (5)	mastocytoma	DBA/2 mouse	methylcholanthrene
YAC (6)	lymphoma	A/Sn mouse	Moloney leukemia v
UV-2237 (7)	fibrosarcoma	C3H⁻ mouse	UV radiation
UV-2237-cl-46 (8)	fibrosarcoma	C3H⁻ mouse	UV radiation
UV-2237 mm (9)	fibrosarcoma	C3H⁻ mouse	UV radiation
K-1735 mm (9)	melanoma	C3H⁻ mouse	UV radiation crotc oil promotio
K-1735 (10)	melanoma	C3H⁻ mouse	UV radiation
3LL (11)	pulmonary carcinoma	$C_{57}BL/6$	unknown
M109 (12, 13)	pulmonary carcinoma	BALB/c	
L1210 (14)	lymphoblastic leukemia	DBA/2	methylcholanthrene
MCA 352 (15)	fibrosarcoma	C_3H	methylcholanthrene
MBL-2 (16)	leukemia	$C_{57}BL/6$	Moloney leukemia v

Tumor lines should be free of mycoplasma and the following pathogenic murine viruses: reovirus type 3, pneumonia virus, K virus, Theiler's encephalitis virus, Sendai virus, minute virus of mice, mouse adenovirus, mouse hepatitis virus, lymphocytic choriomeningitis virus, ectromelia virus, and lactate dehydrogenase virus. Testing can be accomplished commercially by sending specimens to Microbiological Associates, Bethesda, MD.

3.000 IN VIVO TECHNIQUES

3.100 Intravenous Injection

3.101 Standardization of Cell Suspension

The number of tumor cells injected affects lung colony formation; viability and the tumor embolus size and composition can also determine the number of lung colonies formed (17-19). Thus, mice injected with 10,000 clumps of 4-5 cells each developed more

pulmonary foci than did mice injected with 50,000 single tumor
cells. In another study, the injection of 50,000 single cells
yielded an average of 38 pulmonary tumors, whereas the injection
of 50,000 viable tumor cells admixed with 50,000 lethally irradiated
cells yielded 169 tumor foci. Clearly, viability and clump (embolus)
size influences the outcome of experimental metastasis assays. To
avoid clumping of cells, the cell preparations must be free of all
traces of serum, and cells should be injected in a Ca^{++}-and Mg^{++}-free
balanced salt solution, which also serves to decrease clumping (20).

Prolonged (and unnecessary) enzymatic treatment, i.e., trypsinization of tumor cells, can also alter their survival and metastatic
behavior _in vivo_. Moreover, routine viability tests (trypan blue
exclusion) and even plating efficiency _in vitro_ do not predict or
correlate with the _in vivo_ biological behavior of such trypsinized
cells. Trypsinization in excess of 1 min has been reported to decrease lung colony formation and should therefore be avoided (20).

3.102 Intravenous Injection of Tumor Cells

Intravenous injection is the most commonly used route for introducing cells into the circulation. In rats and mice, the lateral
veins in the tail are most often used for intravenous injections.
Dilate the tail vein to facilitate the insertion of a 26- or 27-
gauge needle. Place animals housed in a well-ventilated cage
under a lamp with a 150-W light bulb for 5 min. The distance of
the lamp from the cage can vary, but 4-8 inches is sufficient.
Group the animal by the tail, take it out of the cage, and place
it with its tail protuding through an opening in the wall of a
restraint device. Group the tail between the thumb and the middle
finger, wiped clean with 70% alcohol, and rotate to position the
lateral vein. Stabilized the vein with the index finger. Slight
pressure will straighten the tail and further dilate the lateral
vein. Hold the syringe (0.25 ml, tuberculin type) in the right
hand. A 27-gauge, 3/4-inch needle is most suitable. The bevel
of the needle should always be directed upward. Gently force the
needle through the skin (at a slight angle) and then immediately

thread it (parallel) into the vein. Start the injection slowly; if the needle is not in the vein, tissue resistance to the inoculum can easily be felt. Liquids entering the vein can be visualized during the injection. Intravenous injection of anesthetized mice or of mice that struggle violently should be avoided.

3.103 Enumeration of Pulmonary Tumor Colonies

Tumor colonies that differ in color from the lung parenchyma (melan can be counted with the aid of a dissecting microscope. Mice are killed, and their lungs removed, rinsed in tap water, and fixed in formalin. Extrapulmonary metastases should be noted during necrops and counted. When an organ containing extensive secondary foci is found, it should be removed, rinsed, and fixed for subsequent enume ation of tumor foci. Most pulmonary tumor colonies in mice are in the pleura. Therefore, pigmented colonies (such as melanomas) can be counted without dissection of lungs.

Tumor colonies that are not pigmented and do not differ in color from the pulmonary parenchyma are more difficult to enumerate. The following method is one of several that can be used to induce contrast between tumor colonies and lung parenchyma: Animals suspected of having tumor colonies in their lungs are killed, and thei lungs (or other organs) are removed and rinsed in tap water. A few minutes later, the lungs are placed in a beaker containing Bouin's solution (formaldehyde solution, glacial acetic acid, and a saturated solution of trinitrophenol). The lung parenchyma will immediately turn yellow. Twentyfour hours later, the white tumor colonies will be readily distinguished from the yellow lung parenchyma. The lungs are rinsed in water (to remove excess Bouin's solution), and the tumor colonies are counted with the aid of a dissecting microscope. Murine lungs with greater than 300 colonies should be reported as such (too numerous to count).

3.200 Footpad Injection

Mice to be given injections into a posterior footpad should be restrained by one person while a second person injects the tumor cells. The injection aliquot is 0.05 ml of tumor cells in Ca^{++}-

and Mg^{++}-free HBSS. The leg is grasped at the ankle, and a 3/8-inch, 27-gauge needle is inserted with the bevel up into the proximal side of the central pad. The tight grasp on the ankle and the distal direction of the needle prevent the retroflux movement of tumor cells caused by injection pressure. Make sure that the flow of the injection is toward the nails and not the body.

3.201 Amputation

Mice are lightly anesthetized with methoxyflurane, and the tumor-bearing leg and popliteal lymph node are amputated with a pair of scissors. The wound is rapidly drawn together using wound clips, and the animal is returned to its cage.

3.202 Footpad Measurement

Footpad tumors are to be measured along the two horizontal axes using a vernier caliper. The tumor volume is determined using the formula $0.5 \times a \times b^2$, where a = the larger axis and b = the smaller axis.

3.300 Intraperitoneal Injection

Insert a 25-gauge, 1/2-inch needle into the abdomen, slightly to the side of the site of the umbilicus (a needle inserted below the umbilicus may enter the bladder if the bladder is full). The needle should be inserted, with a stabbing motion, to a depth of not more than 6 mm. Deeper insertion can enter viscera or damage a major blood vessel. The mouse should be released as the needle is withdrawn. Note: Volumes up to 2 ml can easily be inoculated intraperitoneally into mice.

3.400 Subcutaneous Inoculation

Most mice can be successfully inoculated without assistance or anesthesia when the following procedure is adopted:

1. Place the mouse on the metal grid lid of an animal box and hold it by the tail. The animal will grasp the metal rungs; traction on the tail will keep it immobilized.

2. Pick the mouse up by holding the scruff of the neck between the thumb and forefinger of the left hand. Allow its body to fall onto the palm of the hand and catch the base of the tail under the 4th or 5th finger. Move the other fingers under the animal's body so as to stretch the abdominal wall.

3. Direct the 25-gauge, 1/2-inch needle into the pocket of skin lying in the inguinal region. Also make a check to see that the point has not emerged through the skin.

4. Make the injection, then pinch the needle track as the needle is withdrawn in order to close it.

Note: Volumes of 0.1-0.2 ml are suitable for subcutaneous administration.

3.401 Monitoring of Subcutaneous Tumors

Tumors should be measured in two dimensions with use of vernier calipers (see 3.202).

3.500 Intradermal Injection

1. Fill the syringe (0.25 cc syringe) carefully, making sure that no bubbles are trapped in the barrel or needle hub. If any air is present, it will be compressed against the resistance of the dermis to injection, resulting in the delivery of an underdose of the inoculum and also in the deposit of material along the tract of the needle as it is withdrawn, causing leakage.

2. Hold the mouse as one would for a subcutaneous injection and shave the area to be inoculated.

3. Insert the point of the 27-gauge, 1/2-inch needle, bevel uppermost. Force it forward through the skin for about 2 mm. Watch the point of the needle; it should be just visible below th surface.

4. Depress the plunger to inoculate a maximum volume of 0.05 ml.

5. Withdraw the needle and compress the skin along its track with finger and thumb. An inoculation properly placed will blanch the skin as well as produce a persistent, pea-like swelling.

Note: True intradermal inoculations are difficult to achieve in the mouse if volumes that can be measured with an ordinary syringe are injected (use a 0.25 cc syringe). Much of the material is deposited between the dermis proper and the cutaneous muscle lying immediately below it. For these reasons, do not exceed an inoculum volume of 0.05 ml.

3.600 Filling the Syringe

It is desirable (and essential for intradermal or intravenous inoculations) that all air be removed from the barrel of the syringe and from the needle hub. When the inoculum supply is in a sealed vial, this can be easily accomplished. The syringe should be filled and its content emptied back into the vial several times without withdrawal of the needle, until all bubbles have been expurged. When the inoculum is in an open container, the syringe should first be filled with a slightly greater volume of inoculum than that required. The needle should be pointed upwards, and some air should be drawn in until the meniscus can be seen. Next, the barrel should be tapped sharply several times or shaken sharply (as when resetting a clinical thermometer) to make any air bubbles adhering to the walls rise to the top. If the inoculum is very viscous, the plunger should be worked up and down several times while the barrel is viewed against a light. The plunger should be gently pushed up so that the hub and needle fill slowly. As this is done, the hub should be tapped several times to dislodge bubbles. Finally, small quantities of material should be ejected from the needle until no more bubbles are seen.

3.700   Necropsy

1. Kill the mice by administering an overdose of an anesthetic, and pin them onto a cork board.
2. Wet the fur using a cotton swab saturated with 70% ethanol.
3. Make a cut using blunt scissors through the loose skin in the inguinal region and, by blunt dissection, loosen skin to the submandibular region. Reflect the skin until the peritoneum and the thoracic region are widely exposed.
4. Cut through the peritoneum and ribs along the midline, exposing the viscera and thoracic cavity.
5. Remove the lungs, heart, and thymus en bloc.
6. Dissect the heart and float the lungs in water.
7. Fix the lungs in Bouin's solution or formalin.
8. Examine the viscera for grossly visible tumor foci; note the location and extent of any such extrapulmonary foci.
9. Fix suspected extrapulmonary organs in Bouin's solution, and later count the number of tumor foci.
10. Note the location and size, if appropriate, of any lymph node involvement.

11. Measure the size of any primary tumor and/or surgical recurrence in two dimensions using vernier calipers.

12. Note the appearance of any ascites.

3.800 <u>Thymectomy</u>

3.801 Adolescent Mice

Mice 3-4 wk of age and weighing 12-15 g are to be used.

3.801a Reagents

Pentobarbitol anesthesia

70% ethanol

HBSS

3.801b Materials

Autoclips

Autoclip applier

Autoclip remover

Beaker (600-1,000 ml)

Dissecting board

70% ethanol wipes

Lamp to warm mice

1-cc syringes

26-gauge needles

Paper towels

Pasteur pipettes (filed and with flame-polished ends)

Push pins

Recovery cage

Retractor (customized)

Rubber bands

Scale

Scalpel (#10 blades)

Small blunt forceps with serrated edge

Small smooth forceps

Small sharp-pointed scissors (straight)

Suction apparatus consisting of

    flask (1,000 to 1,500-ml Erlenmeyer)

    single-holed rubber stopper for flask

    vacuum tubing (Tygon)

    vacuum source

Tape

3.801c Procedure

1. Set up an aspiration flask by hooking one end of a piece of Tygon tubing to the side arm of an Erlenmeyer flask and the other end of the tubing to a vacuum source. Insert a hollow glass rod through the hole in the rubber stopper and place the stopper in the flask. Attach a 2-ft piece of Tygon tubing to the glass rod. Make a 1-cm hole in the opposite end of the tubing (hole will serve as suction regulator) and attach the specially prepared Pasteur pipette.

2. Set up a dissecting cork board with two push pins inserted in the head side approximately 2 inches apart. Stretch a rubber band over the pins.

3. Weigh the mice and administer 0.01 ml of the diabutal per gram of body weight (less 0.02 ml) intraperitoneally to each of 10 mice. This dose will anesthetized the mice within 5 min.

4. Place a mouse on its back on a dissecting board (covered with an ethanol-saturated paper towel) and immobilize it by hooking the rubber band under its front teeth. Tape the tail down securely and make sure the animal's breathing passage is not obstructed.

5. Swab the neck and chest region with 70% ethanol.

6. Using either a scalpel or scissors, make an incision extending from the xiphoid process to the submandibular region. Reflect the skin edges laterally and pull the salivary gland back toward the head.

7. Staying as close to the midline as possible, carefully insert a blade of the scissors just under the sternum. Make a cut down to the second rib (always point the edge of the scissors upward to ensure that an organ or vessel is not cut).

8. Gently insert the retractor and allow it to spread the chest cavity only enough to expose the thymus.

9. Aspirate the thymus by covering the hole in the tubing with a finger to activate suction and place the tip of the Pasteur pipette on the thymus gland. Pulse the tip up and down until the thymus is completely removed. Clear the Pasteur pipette and suction tubing of thymic tissue by aspirating HBSS through the system.

10. Ascertain that all thymus tissue has been removed. Confirm that all thymic tissue was removed at necropsy. Gently close close the retractor and remove from the chest cavity (move retractor toward you and then up).

11. Quickly close the incision site and autoclip the skin together.

12. Place the mice under a warming lamp (do not overheat) until fully recovered.

13. One week after thymectomy, expose the mice to 800-900 rads whole body irradiation (depending on the strain) and reconstitute the mice with a minimum of 5×10^6 syngeneic bone marrow cells injected intravenously.

14. Four weeks after thymectomy, irradiation, and reconstitution, the animals are ready for study.

3.802 Neonatal Mice

3.802a Materials

Dissecting microscope

Vacuum pump with reservoir

Refrigerator

Adjustable table lamp

Rubber tubing with glass T piece and cannulas

Beaker of detergent solution

Small containers, approximately 20 x 20 x 20 mm; these can be made by cutting up a plastic ice cube tray

Firm bed for newborn mouse. This can be made from a cover-glass container filled with molten wax. When the wax is cool, it can be molded so that the upper surface has a newborn-mouse-shaped hollow

Micropore surgical tape, No. 1530 (Minnesota Mining and Mfg. Co.)

Small cotton-wool swabs, e.g., dental swabs

Nobecutan spray (BDH Pharmaceuticals, Ltd.)

Glass Petri dish

Metal spatula

Iris forceps

Curved iris scissors

Straight iris scissors

Dissecting forceps, fine pointed

3.802b Procedure

1. Hypothermia gives suitable anesthesia for newborn mice. Place the mouse in a small container and put it into the freezer compartment of a refrigerator for 4-5 min.

2. Place the hypothermic mouse supine on the wax bed. Use strips of Micropore tape to hold down the head and limbs, with part of the tape being stuck to the side of the box.

3. Carry out all further manipulations with the aid of a dissecting microscope.

4. Using the forceps, hold the sternum firmly at about the level of the second intercostal space. Then cut across the sternum just below this level (the optimal level for transecting the sternum varies with the strain of mouse).

5. Turn the mouse so that its head is pointed towards or away from you. Hold the cut end of the sternum with the forceps, and enlarge the hole in the chest laterally by blunt dissection. The thymus can be seen under the incision.

6. Remove the thymus by suction, using the same technique described for thymectomy in adult mice.

7. After removal of the thymus, carefully clean away any blood. Replace the flap of skin over the chest wall and reinforce it with a "plastic skin" of Nobecutan: spray some Nobecutan into a glass Petri dish, then pick up a drop with the metal spatula and smear it over the front and sides of the chest.

8. Finally, rewarm the mouse under an electric lamp. When it is warm and moving vigorously, replace it in its mother's cage.

3.900 <u>Bleeding of Mice</u>

3.901 Tail Bleeding

1. Warm the animals under a 150-W light bulb for 5 min.

2. Place the animal in a restraining device with the tail protruding.

3. Wipe the tail clean with a gauze moistened with 70% alcohol.

4. Cut the ventral tail artery with a scaple and rotate the tail slightly to open the incision.

5. Allow the blood to flow into a clean tube.

3.902 Cardiac Puncture

1. Anesthetize a mouse and pin it to a cork board.

2. Wet the fur with 70% ethanol.

3. Make a cut with blunt scissors through the loose skin in the inguinal region and, by blunt dissection, loosen the skin to the submandibular region. Reflect skin so the thoracic region is exposed.

4. Cut through the ribs, exposing the heart without nicking a maj blood vessel or the heart.

5. Insert a 25-gauge needle attached to a 1-ml syringe into a ven ricle and slowly exsanguinate the mouse (0.5-1.0 ml per mouse)

6. Remove the needle and place the blood into a centrifuge tube.

7. Allow the blood to clot at room temperature for 5 min.

8. Rim the blood clot and allow the clot to retract on ice for 30

9. Centrifuge and carefully remove the serum.

10. Sterilize the serum using a syringe and a filter (0.22 micron)

11. Freeze, or store at 4°C.

3.903 Subaxillary Bleeding

1. Anesthetize a mouse, and pin it to a cork board.

2. Wet the fur with 70% ethanol.

3. Make a cut through the skin over the xiphoid process and loose the skin by blunt dissection dorsally.

4. Reflect the skin in such a manner as to form a pocket in the s axillary region.

5. Snip the brachial artery and allow blood to pool in the pocket formed by the skin.

6. Collect the blood using a Pasteur pipette and place it into a centrifuge tube.

7. Allow the blood to clot at room temperature for 5 min and then rim the clot.

8. Allow the clot to retract on ice for 30 min.

9. Centrifuge and carefully remove the serum.

10. Sterilize the serum using a syringe and a filter (0.22 micron)

11. Freeze, or store at 4°C.

3.904 Puncture of the Retro - Orbital Plexus

1. Lightly anesthetize the animal.

2. Grasp the animal by the skin at the back of the neck and hold

securely to a flat surface.

3. Pull the loose skin on the head and adjacent to the eye taut so that the eye protrudes slightly from its socket.

4. Moisten a Pasteur pipette, fitted with a suction bulb, with heparin.

5. Insert the end into the orbital cavity at the lower inside corner of the eye. Slide it in parallel to the eye to the ophthalmic venous plexus at the back of the orbit.

6. Withdraw the tip slightly. The blood will fill the pipette by capillary action, which can be aided by the suction bulb.

7. Quantities of 1 ml can be obtained from mice in this manner.

8. Bleeding stops quickly when the pipette is removed. If small quantities are obtained this is a survival procedure.

4.000 TISSUE CULTURE PROTOCOLS

4.100 Reagents

EMEM

DMSO

FBS

Gentamicin

Kanamycin

HEPES

NEAA

EAA

Nucleic acid stock, 100X stock solution

Williams medium E

EMEM (methionine free)

Sodium bicarbonate, 7.5%

MEM vitamins, 100X solution

L-Glutamine, 200 mM

Sodium pyruvate, 100 mM

2-ME

RPMI-1640 medium

HBSS

10X HBSS

CMF-HBSS

4.200 Preparation of Tissue Culture Medium

4.201 Complete Minimum Essential Medium (CMEM)

	Volume (ml)
EMEM	500
Sodium bicarbonate (if required)	15
MEM vitamins	10
L-Glutamine	5
NEAA	5
Sodium pyruvate	5
Gentamicin (assays only)	0.5
FBS	25 (5%) or 50 (10%)

4.202 Complete EMEM (methionine free)

EMEM (methionine free)	500
L-Glutamine	5
Gentamicin	0.5
FBS (not heat inactivated)	25

4.203 Complete Williams medium E

Williams medium E	500
Sodium pyruvate	5
L-Glutamine	5
Gentamicin (assays only)	0.5
FBS	100 (17%)

4.204 Complete RPMI-1640

RPMI-1640	500
L-Glutamine	5
Gentamicin	0.5
ΔFBS	25

4.205 Extra high amino acids (EHAA) medium (21, 22, 23)

Medium (listed in the order in which it is added)

Stock ingredient	Stock (per 100 ml EHAA)
Sterile distilled H_2O	64.0 ml
HBSS (10X)	10.0 ml
EMEM EAA (50X)	5.0 ml
EMEM NEAA (100X)	4.0 ml
EMEM vitamins (100X)	2.0 ml
Sodium pyruvate (100 mm)	2.5 ml
L-Glutamine (200 mm)	2.0 ml
Nucleic acid precursors (100X)	2.5 ml
NaOH 2 N to pH 7-7.4	~ 0.5 ml
Gentamicin	0.1 ml

Adjust the pH to 7-7.4, by using a sterile Pasteur pipette and litmus paper to maintain a sterile source. The above mixture 1X EHAA can be stored at -20°C until use. Before use, add the following per 100 ml EHAA:

2-ME (0.1 M)	0.04 ml
Sodium bicarbonate (7.5%)	1.8 ml

4.205a Stock nucleic acid precursors (100X)

Adenosine	1 g
Cytosine	1 g
Guanosine	1 g
Uridine	1 g
Distilled water	1 liter distilled H_2O

Filter, sterilize, and store at 4°C.

4.205b Preparation of normal mouse serum (NMS)

(see section 3.901)

4.206 Medium for P815

Minimum essential medium	500 ml
L-Glutamine	5 ml
FBS	50 ml
MEM vitamins	10 ml
NEAA	5 ml
Sodium pyruvate	5 ml

4.300 Cell Cryopreservation Medium

Stock (to be used ice cold)	Volume (ml)
EMEM - supplemented (exactly as described above)	325
ΔFBS	125
DMSO (sterilize by autoclaving)	50

Note: Prepare fresh as needed. Do not store.

4.400 Preparation of Assay Reagents

4.401 $[^{125}I]$IUdR

Dilute 1 ml of $[^{125}I]$IUdR (1 mCi/ml stock) in 99 ml of CMF-HBSS and pass the solution through a bacteriological filter. Check activity by counting 0.01 ml on a gamma counter (expected count range, 100,000-200,000 cpm). Final $[^{125}I]$IUdR stock = 10 μCi/ml. Store refrigerated.

4.402 $[^3H]$Proline, 1 mCi/ml stock (20-40 Ci/mmol). Store refrigerated.

4.403 $[^{75}Se]$Methionine

Dilute stock in methionine-free CMEM and 5% FBS to 10 μCi/ml. Store refrigerated.

4.404 $[^3H]$Thymidine

Dilute $[^3H]$thymidine stock (2 Ci/mmol, 1 mCi/ml), 1:25 in sterile H to obtain a final concentration of 40 μCi/ml. When labeling with 1 μCi/well, add 0.025 ml of the diluted stock. Store refrigerated.

4.405 1% Triton X-100

Dissolve 1 ml of Triton X-100 in 99 ml of sterile distilled water. Store at room temperature.

4.406 2% Sodium Dodecyl Sulfate (SDS)

Dissolve 2 g SDS in 100 ml sterile distilled water. Store at room temperature.

4.407 0.1 M Sodium Hydroxide (NaOH)

Dissolve 4 g NaOH in 1,000 ml sterile distilled water and add a sli amount of methylene blue as a marker. Store at room temperature. Note: caustic material.

4.408 White Blood Cell Counting Fluid (WBCF)

Add 3.0 ml glacial acetic acid and 0.01 g methyl violet to 100 ml d tilled water. Mix thoroughly and filter. Store at room temperature

4.409 Trypan Blue Stain (0.4%)

Dilute the trypan blue stain 1:2 in sterile saline so as to obtain a final stock concentration of 0.2%. Dilute cell suspensions in 0.2% trypan blue stock prior to performing a hemacytometer count. Store at room temperature.

4.410 Mitomycin C

Dissolve mitomycin C in sterile HBSS at a concentration of 0.5 mg/ml (4 ml HBSS/2 mg vial). Store refrigerated and protected from light. If a precipitate forms on storage, discard and prepare fresh reagent. Prepare fresh reagent weekly.

4.411 2-Mercaptoethanol (2-ME)

Caution: 2-ME is extremely toxic and malodorous. Perform all dilutions in a chemical fume hood.

Make a 1.0 M solution of 2-ME (Sigma #M-6250, density = 1.114 g/ml, molarity = 14.3 M) by diluting 0.5 ml 2-ME into 6.6 ml sterile distilled water. Dilute 20 ml of the 1.0 M stock into 90 ml of sterile water to give a concentration of 1×10^{-1} M. Store refrigerated.

4.412 Trypsin-EDTA Solution

Dilute 20 ml of 10X trypsin-EDTA solution with 100 ml CMF-HBSS to give a working solution.

4.413 Phosphate-Buffered Saline-Tween (PBS-Tween), pH 7.4, 1 liter

NaCl, 8.0 g

KH_2PO_4 (potassium phosphate monobasic), 0.2 g

Na_2HPO_4 (anh. sodium phosphate), 1.15 g

KCl (potassium chloride), 0.2 g

Tween-80, 0.5 ml

NaN_3 (sodium azide), 0.2 g

Bring volume to 1 liter. Store at 4°C for 2 weeks.

4.414 Carbonate Coating Buffer, pH 9.8, 1 liter

Na_2CO_3 (sodium carbonate anh.), 1.59 g

$NaHCO_3$ (sodium bicarbonate), 2.93 g

NaN_3 (sodium azide), 0.2 g

Bring to 1 liter. Make up fresh daily.

4.415 10% Diethanolamine Buffer, 1 liter

Diethanolamine, 97 ml, if in liquid form. If not, weigh out to 10% final concentration.

distilled H_2O, 800 ml

NaN_3, - 0.2 g

$MgCl_2$.$6H_2O$, 100 mg

Bring pH to 9.8 with 1 M HCl. Store at 4°C in the dark. Remove sufficient amount 1 to 2 before the substrate solution is to be used and allow it to warm to room temperature. Keeps for 3 months. Should be kept in the dark in brown bottle.

4.416 Substrate Solution

1 Sigma tablet = 5 mg in 5 ml 10% diethanolamine

or powder = 1 mg in 1 ml 10% diethanolamine (need 10 ml total/ plate)

4.500 Harvesting of Adherent Tumor Cells

1. Split cells 48 hr before using.
2. Refeed cells 24 hr before harvesting.
3. Pour off culture medium from adherent cell monolayers.
4. Add trypsin-EDTA solution to the tissue culture flask (7 ml/T-1 flask; 3 ml/T-75 flask), gently overlay the monolayer, and immediately remove excess solution with pipette.
5. Place tissue culture flask on a flat surface (monolayer side down) and wait 60 sec. Tap the flask sharply to dislodge the adherent cells.
6. Once the cells have dislodged, add at least 10 ml of CMEM-FBS to each flask.
7. Pool the harvested cells into 50-ml centrifuge tubes, fill the tubes with CMEM-FBS, and centrifuge at 1,000 rpm for 5 min.
8. Wash cells 1X in CMF-HBSS and resuspend in a small volume of the appropriate physiological medium.
9. Perform a viable cell count in trypan blue stain and adjust the viable cell concentration to the number desired per milliliter in the appropriate physiological medium.

Note: Tumor cells that are to be injected _in vivo_ should be washed 2X in CMF-HBSS before counting and injection.

4.600 Radiolabeling of Tumor Cells

4.601 [^{125}I]IUdR Labeling

1. Twenty-four hours prior to labeling tumor cells, split cells from a confluent 75-cm^2 tissue culture flask 1:3 as described in section 4.500.

2. One day prior to labeling cells, refeed T-75 flask with 10 ml of fresh medium.

3. Label cells by refeeding cells with 10 ml fresh medium (10% FBS) containing 0.2-0.3 ml of [^{125}I]IUdR stock (10 µCi/ml) to each 75-cm^2 tissue culture flask.

Note: Target cells should be in log growth phase at the time label is added. Each target line grows at a slightly different rate. Adjust dilution at time of split accordingly.

4. On the following day (24 hr after label addition), harvest target cells as described in section 4.500. Wash monolayer 2X with warm HBSS to remove nonbound radioiodine before trypsinization. Perform a cell count in trypan blue and adjust cells to the required number.

5. Determine input counts of labeled target cells by adding 0.2 ml of the labeled cell suspension to a 12 x 75-mm glass tube. Place tube in gamma counter and determine input cpm.

Note: Input cpm/1 x 10^4 labeled cells should be at least 1,500. If labeling is higher than 0.5 to 1.0 cpm per cell, radiotoxicity could occur. Furthermore, if labeling were greater than 1.0 cpm/cell and cells were labeled in 0.3-0.5 µCi [^{125}I]IUdR/ml culture medium, one should suspect Mycoplasma contamination.

4.602 [^{3}H]Proline Labeling

1. One day before labeling cells with [^{3}H]proline, split cells into a T-75 tissue culture flask so as to obtain a 40%-50% confluent monolayer culture 24 hr later.

2. Twenty-four hours after splitting the cells, wash the monolayer culture with medium devoid of NEAA. Add 0.15 ml of [^{3}H]proline stock and 10 ml of medium devoid of nonessential amino acids to the T-75 flask monolayer culture and incubate for 24 hr.

3. Harvest [^{3}H]proline-labeled cells as described in section 4.500.

4. Wash and resuspend the cells.

5. Perform a cell count and adjust cells to the required number.

6. Determine input counts of labeled target cells by solubilizing 10^4 labeled cells in 0.2 ml of 1% Triton X. Transfer the Triton-X-solubilized cell mixture to scintillation fluid. Determine cpm in a beta counter.

Note: Input cpm/10^4 labeled cells should be at least 5,000.

4.603 ^{51}Cr Labeling

1. Use actively growing (log phase) cells (at least 90% viable).

2. Wash cells and suspend 5×10^6 cells in 0.3 ml medium.

3. Add 200 µCi of ^{51}Cr in a volume of 0.2 ml (100 µCi/0.1 ml of stock) to a 15-ml conical bottom tube containing 5×10^6 cells; gently mix the cells and chromium together.

4. Incubate cells at 37°C in a water bath for 45 min (YAC-1) or 60 min (P815). Every 10-15 min, gently resuspend cells.

5. After incubation, bring volume of Cr-labeled cells to 10 ml with medium.

6. Centrifuge cells at 1,200 rpm for 6 min. Wash cells twice in at least 10 ml of medium.

7. Gently resuspend cells in 10 ml medium and incubate at 37°C in a water bath for 15 min.

8. Centrifuge cells at 1,200 rpm for 6 min. Gently resuspend cells in 5 ml medium, perform a cell count, and adjust the cell concentration.

Note: If Cr-labeled cells cannot be used immediately, store on ice.

9. Determine input counts by measuring cpm present in 0.1 ml of the Cr-labeled cell suspension (test in triplicate).

4.604 ^{111}In Labeling (Indium Oxine)

1. Use actively growing (log phase) cells (at least 90% viable).

2. Wash cells and suspend 10×10^6 cells in 0.5 ml medium.

3. Add 15 µCi of ^{111}In to a 50-ml conical bottom tube containing 10×10^6 cells; gently mix the cells and indium together. Due to the very short half-life of ^{111}In, the specific activity should be calculated daily (see appendix).

4. Incubate cells at 37°C in a water bath for 10-15 min.

5. After incubation, bring volume of ^{111}In-labeled cells to 50 ml with medium.

6. Centrifuge cells at 1,200 rpm for 6 min. Wash cells twice in at least 50 ml of medium and adjust the cell concentration.

Note: If ^{111}In-labeled cells cannot be used immediately, store on ice.

7. Determine input counts by measuring cpm present in 0.1 ml of the cell ^{111}In-labeled suspension (test in triplicate).

4.700 <u>Cryopreservation of Cells</u> (may also use a controlled rate freezer)

1. Collect adherent tumor cells as described under section 4.500 or collect suspension-grown tumor cells by centrifugation. (Keep cells on ice throughout processing.)

2. Wash the cells 1X in CMEM-5% FBS and resuspend in an appropriate volume of CMEM-5% FBS.

3. Perform a viable cell count using trypan blue stain.

4. Prelabel the appropriate number of Nunc vials with an alcohol-resistant marker with cell name and date.

5. Centrifuge the cells at 1,200 rpm for 6 min and resuspend in cold cryopreservation medium at a concentration of 2-10 x 10^6 viable cells/ml. Store on ice.

6. Apportion 1 ml of the cells in cryopreservation medium/into NUNC or comprable vessel. Keep on ice.

7. Place all Nunc vials at -20°C until frozen.

8. Immediately transfer the vials to -70°C for approximately 16 hr.

9. Transfer the vials to the vapor phase of a liquid nitrogen freezer for long-term storage.

10. Record the cell name, number per milliliter, date, number of vials frozen, and location within the liquid nitrogen freezer in the freezer log book.

11. Remove a sample vial from the liquid nitrogen freezer 7 days after freezing and thaw rapidly in a 37°C water bath.

12. As soon as cells are thawed, place the cells into a T-75 flask. Drop by drop (very slowly to avoid osmotic shock), add 10 ml serum containing medium.

13. Slowly add an additional 30 ml with serum to dilute medium the DMSO.

14. Incubate 37°C for 24 hr.

15. Remove medium containing DMSO and refeed with routine amount of medium-FBS.

4.800 Mitomycin C Treatment of Cells (24)

1. Prepare the cell suspension in HBSS at a concentration of 1×10^7 cells/ml in a 15-ml conical-bottom centrifuge tube.

2. Add 25 µg of mitomycin C (0.05 ml of 0.5 mg/ml stock) per milliliter of cell suspension.

3. Incubate cells in mitomycin C mixture for 30 min in a 37°C water bath with gentle mixing every 10 min; protect the incubating mixture from light.

4. Wash cells 3X in 10 ml of CMEM + 5% ΔFBS.

5. Perform a cell count and adjust the cells to the number desired per milliliter in appropriate assay medium.

4.900 Heat Inactivation of FBS

1. Remove FBS from freezer.

2. Thaw overnight in refrigerator.

3. Bring to 37°C in a water bath.

4. Submerge in 56°C water that reaches the level of the top of the serum for 30 min.

5. Shake bottles well.

6. Store at 4°C or freeze.

4.1000 Establishment of a Primary Tumor Culture

1. Kill the mice by administering an overdose of anesthetic.

2. Submerge mice in an iodine solution.

3. Submerge mice in 70% ethanol.

4. Pin mice onto a towel (saturated with 70% ethanol) on a cork board. Place the board into a laminar airflow hood.

5. Make a cut using sterile instruments (set 1) through the loose skin in the inguinal region and extend by blunt dissection to the submandibular region. Carefully reflect the skin by blunt dissection away from a subcutaneous tumor.

6. Wash the tumor and peritoneum using 70% ethanol.

7. Dissect out the tumor, or open the mouse, with a second set of sterile instruments.

8. Place tumor tissue into a tissue culture plate containing sterile CMF-HBSS (2X gentamicin).
9. Remove necrotic tissue and any adherent normal tissue.
10. Place the tumor tissue in a second vessel containing CMF-HBSS 2X gentamicin. Mince the tissue into 1-mm fragements using crossed scalpel blades.
11. Remove the fragments and wash in CMEM.
12. Place the minced tissue in a 100-mm tissue culture plate, feed with an appropriate medium, and culture at 37°C.

4.1100 General Toxicity Assay

1. Use actively growing (log phase) target cells.
2. Gently trypsinize target cells.
3. Wash the target cells and suspend at 1×10^3 cells/ml in Ca^{++}-Mg^{++} free HBSS (single cell suspension). Predetermine the clonal plating efficiency and add cells sufficient to result in ~100 colonies.
4. Use one six-well plate (30 mm in diameter) for each test group.
5. Add 5 ml of medium to each well.
6. Add 100 microliters of the suspended tumor cell to each well, using a repeating pipette aid.
7. After adding the cells to a plate, agitate the medium to evenly suspend the cells.
8. Incubate the plates for 4 hr.
9. Add the drugs or diluent in a 100 microliter volume at a concentration to result in the desired dose (minimum of five doses per drug).
10. Gently mix the medium-drug.
11. Incubate for a predetermined interval (12-24 hr) at 37°C.
12. Aspirate the drug containing medium and wash the wells twice with complete medium.
13. Refeed the cultures with complete medium.
14. Incubate the plates 8-12 days (until 1- to 3-mm diameter colonies are formed).
15. Aspirate the medium.
16. Fix and stain target cell colonies using a saturated solution of methylene blue in a 50% aqueous-methanol solution.

4.1200 Growth Curves

1. Use actively growing (log phase) cells.
2. Gently trypsinize cells.
3. Wash the cells and suspend at 1×10^6 cells/ml in Ca^{++}- Mg^{++}-free HBSS as a single cell suspension.
4. Add 5 ml of complete medium to 35 culture dishes (60-mm) per cell line.
5. Add 100 microliters of cells (10^5 cells) to each 60-mm dish.
6. Immediately agitate the dish to evenly suspend the tumor cells.
7. Incubate the cells at 37°C.
8. Feed cells two times per week.
9. Count the number of cells per dish (in triplicate) on days 1, 2, 3, 4, 7, 9, 11, 14, 16, and 18 or until a plateau is reached (schedule days correctly - 1, 2, 3, 4, and 7 are critical ones)
10. To count the number of cells per dish:
    a) Aspirate the medium from three dishes.
    b) Add 3 ml trypsin to each dish.
    c) Wait until all cells have detached (you may wish to agitate the trypsin-cells several times).
    d) Remove all medium and cells (measure to 0.1 ml the amount).
    e) Dilute cells in an exact amount of dilution buffer.
    f) Aspirate through the Coulter counter (count each sample 3X) If several samples are being counted, store vials on ice.
    g) Record cell counts.
11. Set 35 plates - the 5 extras will allow for some loss due to contamination or for additional time points if a plateau is not reached by day 18. If after three readings the cell counts have not increased or have decreased (assuming saturation density and not toxicity), discontinue the assay.

5.000 QUALITY CONTROL

5.100 Testing of Media

One representative 500-ml bottle of medium from each production lot should be subjected to the following tests:

1. Microbial contamination: Filter two 150-ml aliquots of each type of medium through 25-mm bacteriological disc filters.

Place the filters in 150 ml of thioglycolate and trypticase soy broth, respectively. Incubate the broths at 37°C for 48 hr and examine for microbial growth.

2. Endotoxin content: A qualitative and quantitative <u>Limulus</u> amebocyte lysate assay is performed. (see 5:300)

Before a given lot of medium is used in a preclinical screen; The medium must meet the following criteria:

Be free of microbial contamination.

Be free of endotoxin.

Support clonal cell growth.

Not activate NK cells <u>in vitro</u> or <u>in vivo</u>.

Not inhibit effector cell functions.

5.200 <u>Testing of Sera</u>

One representative 500-ml bottle of FBS from each lot should be subjected to the following tests.

1. Microbial contamination: Filter two 150-ml aliquots from each serum lot through 25-mm bacteriological disc filters. Place the filters in 150 ml of thioglycolate and trypticase soy broth, respecfively. Incubate the broths at 37°C for 48 hr and examine for microbial growth.

2. Testing for <u>Mycoplasma</u>: Inoculate serum of E agar and into diphasic E broth (alternative assays are also available).

3. Endotoxin content: Perform a qualitative and quantitative <u>Limulus</u> amebocyte lysate assay (see 5:300).

Before a given lot of serum is used in the preclinical screen; The serum must meet the following criteria:

Be free of microbial contamination.

Be free of <u>Mycoplasma</u> organisms.

Support clonal cell growth.

Not inhibit effector cell functions.

5.300 <u>Testing for the Presence of Endotoxin</u> (25)

5.301 Reagents and Materials

The <u>Limulus</u> amebocyte lysate (Pyrotell) Single Vial Test Kit (Associates of Cape Cod, Inc.).

5.302   Procedure

As described in the Pyrotell test kit manual.

In summary:

Limulus amebocyte lysate assay is employed to detect endotoxin contamination in various solutions. The assay is rapid and specific and can detect subnanogram quantities of endotoxin per milliliter. To perform the test, 0.2 ml of test sample (various dilutions in endotoxin-free medium) is added to a blue color-coded 12 x 75-mm tube that contains 0.2 ml freeze-dried lysate. After mixing, the tube is incubated undisturbed in a 37°C water bath for 1 hr. A positive test is indicated by the formation of a gel that does not collapse upon 180° inversion of the test tube. A quantitative estimate of the amount of endotoxin in samples can be made by performing serial dilutions of samples along with dilutions of a standard endotoxin preparation and determining at what concentration of endotoxin a positive test is no longer obtained. Standard endotoxin preparations must always be carried out in parallel with test samples to confirm the sensitivity of the assay.

5.400   Contamination of Cell Lines

All cell lines need to be examined for the presence of contagious murine viruses and Mycoplasma organisms. The murine viruses are examined by the use of the MAP test by Microbiological Associates (Bethesda, MD) and include reovirus type 3, pneumonia virus of mice, K virus, Theiler's virus, Sendai virus, minute virus, mouse adenovirus, mouse hepatitis virus, lymphocytic choriomeningitis virus, ectromelia virus, and lactate dehydrogenase virus.

All cell lines must be examined for the presence of viruses twice a year and are maintained as antibiotic-free stock cultures. On a bimonthly basis, all the cell lines are examined for bacterial and Mycoplasma contamination and reinitiated from frozen stocks.

5.500   Testing of [^{125}I]IUdR Stock

1. Split the appropriate tumor target cells 24 hr before the addition of [^{125}I]IUdR to the cultures so that the cells are in log phase growth at the time the [^{125}I]IUdR label is added.

2. Harvest the cells from a confluent 75-cm^2 tissue culture flask as described under section 4.500 and split 1:4 into four additional 75-cm^2 tissue culture flasks containing 10 ml of CMEM.

3. Twenty-four hours later, add 0.2, 0.4, or 0.6 ml of the new [^{125}I]IUdR stock (10 μCi/ml) or 0.3 ml of the old [^{125}I]IUdR stock to flasks.

4. Incubate the cells with the [^{125}I]IUdR stock for an additional 24 hr. Harvest and plate a minimum of three wells/cell group (add 10^4 cells per well) as described in section 14.300.

5. Harvest triplicate wells of each of the labeled cell lines 24 and 72 hr after plating as described in section 14.400.

Note: A new stock is suitable for use if it is not toxic as measured by the ability of the labeled target cells to adhere and to retain their radioactive label and the ability to proliferate in vitro 72 hr after plating.

6.000 CELLULAR PREPARATIONS EX VIVO

6.100 Preparation of Lymphoid Cell Suspensions
(Suitable for spleen, thymus, or lymph node)

6.101 Reagents
70% ethanol
10X HBSS
Sterile distilled water
RPMI-1640 medium + gentamicin
Trypan blue stain

6.102 Materials
Small glass beaker
Dissecting boards
Paper towels
Blunt scissors
Toothed forceps
Pointed scissors
Serrated forceps
100-mm Petri dishes
Sterile 80 mesh tissue sieves

Sterile 5-cc syringe plungers

Sterile nylon boltex cloth sieve

Ice

Ice bucket

50-ml conical-bottom centrifuge tubes

12 x 75-mm glass tubes

1-, 5-, 10-ml pipettes; Pasteur pipettes

Hemacytometer

Compound research microscope

Refrigerated centrifuge (Beckman TJ-6)

6.103   Procedure

1.   Set up the following in a laminar airflow hood:

A beaker of 95% ethanol containing the scissors and forceps

An ice bucket containing 50-ml tubes

100-mm Petri dishes

Animal dissection cord board covered with an ethanol-saturat

paper towel

2.   Kill the mice by cervical dislocation.

3.   Wash the mice in an iodine solution and then in 70% ethanol.
Place the mice onto a clean towel with their left sides up.

4.   Saturate the mice with ethanol. Cut with blunt scissors throug
the loose skin in the inguinal region, and reflect skin toward
the head and tail until the peritoneum is widely exposed.

5.   Lavage the skin with 70% ethanol.

6.   Lift the peritoneal wall over the spleen with toothed forceps
and make a large U-shaped cut with blunt scissors around the
spleen. Fold back the peritoneum; lift the spleen with the
serrated forceps and separate it from the vessels and connectiv
tissue with the pointed scissors. Place the spleens from each
experimental group into a 100-mm Petri dish containing 8-10
ml of cold RPMI-1640 medium.

7.   Place the spleens into a tissue sieve and cut each spleen into
three pieces. Using a plunger of a 5-cc syringe, press the
spleen pieces through the stainless steel grid to obtain single
cells and aggregates. Aspirate the cell suspension up and
down in a 10-ml pipette to break up any large aggregates.

8. Filter the cell suspension through a nylon mesh sieve into a 50-ml tube on ice. Add approximately 40 ml of RPMI-1640 medium to the tube and centrifuge the cells at 1,200 rpm for 6 min.

9. Water lyse the red blood cells in the following manner. Resuspend the cell pellet in 9 ml of sterile distilled water (3-5 sec), vortex, immediately add 1 ml of sterile 10X HBSS, and vortex.

10. Remove cell debris by filtering the cell suspension through another nylon sieve.

11. Wash the cells once in RPMI-1640 medium. After the final centrifugation at 1,200 rpm for 6 min, resuspend the cells in the appropriate assay medium and perform a cell count in trypan blue stain. Adjust the cells to the number of desired viable cells per milliliter and store on ice.

6.200 Collection of Mouse Peritoneal Cells (Resident Macrophages)

6.201 Reagents

95% ethanol

Trypan blue

CMF-HBSS + 2X gentamicin

WBCF

6.202 Materials

5-cc syringes

22-gauge needles

Blunt scissors

Toothed forceps

1-, 5-, 10-ml pipettes; Pasteur pipettes

50-ml conical-bottom centrifuge tubes

10 x 75-mm glass tubes

Dissecting boards

Paper towels

100-ml glass beaker

Ice

Ice bucket

Hemacytometer

Compound research microscope

Refrigerated centrifuge (Beckman TJ-6)

6.203 Procedure

1. Set up the following in a horizontal laminar airflow hood:
    100-ml sterile beaker filled with CMF-HBSS + 2X gentamicin
    Ice bucket containing 50-ml tubes
    Dissection board covered with an ethanol-saturated paper towel
    Pair of blunt scissors and toothed forceps

2. Kill the mice by inhalation anesthesia overdose.

3. Wash mice in an iodine solution, then again in 70% ethanol.

4. Place the mice ventral side up on a dissection board.

5. Swab the abdominal area with alcohol and make a small cut
    through the skin in the inguinal region. Be careful not to
    puncture the abdominal wall.

6. Secure the tail with one hand and reflect the skin back with
    the other hand so as to expose the peritoneum, then pin the
    animal. Wash the mice with 70% ethanol.

7. Fill a 10-cc syringe with 6-8 ml of CMF-HBSS + 2X gentamicin
    and aseptically attach a 20 to 22-gauge needle.

8. Carefully insert the needle into the midline of the peritoneum,
    taking care not to puncture any organ. Inject the fluid and
    withdraw the needle. Recap the needle and syringe and place
    the needle end of the syringe in an elevated position.

9. Gently agitate the abdominal cavity by moving the board to
    which the animals are pinned.

10. Reinsert the needle into the peritoneum at a site adjucent
    to the kidney and slowly aspirate out the fluid. If the
    needle becomes obstructed, remove it and reinsert in another
    area. Collect a total of 5 ml of fluid.

11. Aseptically remove the needle from the syringe and transfer
    the fluid into a 50-ml tube. Store on ice.

12. Repeat steps 4-8 two more times. The fluid recovery from
    each of the washes should be 4 ml or more.

13. Centrifuge the cells at 1,200 rpm for 6 min in a refrigerated
    centrifuge.

14. Resuspend the cell pellet in the appropriate assay medium.
    Make a dilution and perform a total cell count in WBCF.

15. Adjust the cells to the desired number per milliliter.

16. Keep all cells on ice throughout the collection procedure and until plated.

6.300 <u>Collection of Mouse Peritoneal Exudate Cells (Thioglycolate Elicited)</u>

Inject 1 ml of fluid thioglycolate/10 g body weight i.p. into each mouse 5 or 6 days prior to peritoneal lavage.

Peritoneal lavage (see 6.201, 6.202, and 6.203).

6.400 <u>Collection of Rat Alveolar Macrophages</u>

6.401 Reagents

95% and 70% ethanol

Sodium pentobarbital

CMF - HBSS

Gentamicin (50 mg/ml stock)

6.402 Materials

1-cc tuberculin syringe

5-cc syringes

19- and 22-gauge needles

19- or 21-gauge butterfly infusion sets (Abbott Labs)

Dissecting boards

Paper towels

2 small pointed scissors

1 large curved scissors

2 large toothed forceps

Carpet thread

100-mm Petri dishes

250-ml conical-bottom centrifuge tubes (Corning #25350)

Glass beaker

125-ml trypsinizing flask

Ice

Ice bucket

37°C water bath thermometer

Sterile gauze pads

Refrigerated centrifuge

Bunsen burner

Rats, 12-16 wk of age

6.403 Procedure

1. Set up the following in a horizontal laminar airflow hood:

   37°C water bath

   Bunsen burner

   Beaker of 95% ethanol containing scissors and forceps

2. Using sterile technique, insert a 19-gauge butterfly unit into the side arm of a 125-ml trypsinizing flask as follows: Hold the butterfly unit by the hub end and cut at the second major curve in the tubing (approximately 16 cm long). Discard the needle end. Grasping the plastic hub with your fingers, stretch the tubing taut with forceps and insert into the trypsinizing flask.

3. Add 1 ml gentamicin per 500 ml of prewarmed (37°C) HBSS. Transfer the solution to the prepared trypsinizing flask and place it in a water bath (37°C).

4. Place an ice bucket in the hood with the appropriate number of 250-ml tubes (generally one tube per treatment group of three rats).

5. Cut carpet thread to a length of 6 inch for each rat.

6. Cut the Luer lock tips from the ends of the 5-cc syringes (one syringe per rat to be lavaged) and place the syringes in a sterile Petri dish.

7. Prepare butterfly units (19-gauge for large rats and 21-gauge for small rats) for lavage by cutting the tubing 2 cm from the hub end and discarding the remaining tubing and needle. Place the prepared butterfly units in a sterile Petri dish.

8. Anesthetize the rats by injecting sodium pentobarbital i.p. (30 mg/kg body weight or approximately 0.3 ml/rat). Within 5 min, the rats should be anesthetized and can be pinned to the dissecting boards (covered with ethanol-saturated paper towels), ventral side up. Disinfect the entire ventral side with 70% ethanol.

9. Reflect the peritoneum and exsanguinate the rats by severing one or both renal arteries. (This procedure minimizes post-mortem pulmonary edema and reduces the amount of blood trapped in the lungs.)

10. Reflect the skin from the chest area by a straight central cut from the liver to the chin.

11. Carefully dissect out the salivary gland, exposing the trachea. Try not to sever blood vessels on either side of the salivary gland.

12. Open the chest cavity from the anterior end of the rib cage by making a straight midline cut down the sternum, exposing the lungs and heart. Be sure not to cut the lungs or heart. Carefully cut away the rib cage on either side of the lungs, leaving about 1 cm of the rib cage.

Note: Perform the following techniques under sterile conditions in the hood.

13. Remove the membrane surrounding the trachea. Cannulate the trachea in the following manner: Insert a pair of forceps under the trachea and raise it slightly. Make a small perpendicular cut in the trachea at a point three fourths of the distance up the exposed trachea (away from the lungs). Lift the forceps higher, causing the cut to gape. Insert the precut butterfly tube into the trachea as far as possible; anchor it securely with carpet thread encircling the trachea and tie it off.

14. Place a sterile gauze pad under the hub of the butterfly tubing so as to keep the area sterile.

15. Attach a 5-cc syringe containing 4 cc of warm CMF-HBSS to the hub of each infusion set in each trachea. (The angle of the syringe when attached to the hub of the infusion set is very important. Preserve the natural curve of the tubing. Failure to do so will result in blockage of the trachea either by the tubing or in suction of the trachea wall into the tubing.)

Note: Do the lavage in an assembly line fashion, i.e. lavage several rats sequentially. Six rats is the maximum number of rats that should be lavaged by one person at one time.

16. Aspirate the air from the lungs by withdrawing the syringe plunger 1 cc. Slowly inject 1 cc at a time into each lung until only 1 cc remains in each syringe. Inject the remaining 1 cc and immediately aspirate out the fluid from the lung. Expected yield

is 3 cc with 1 cc remaining in the areola of the lung.

17. Transfer the aspirated fluid into a 250-ml collection vessel on ice. Refill the syringe with 5 cc of CMF-HBSS, reattach the infusion tubing, and inject 4 cc into each lung. Allow this volume of fluid to sit in the lung until the infusion is complete for each rat.

18. Inject the remaining 1 cc of CMF-HBSS and immediately aspirate the fluid from the lungs, recovering approximately 5 cc. Transfer fluid into a 250-ml collection tube set in ice.

19. Infuse fluid repeatedly as described in steps 16 and 17. However this time, aspirate out 3 cc into the syringe and immediately reinject int, then aspirate out 5 cc of fluid and transfer it into a 250-ml collection vessel set in ice.

Repeat lavage procedure until desired volume is obtained.

Suggested ecovery volume: 2 rats = 150 ml

3 rats = 250 ml

Expected yield per rat of 200 grams: $3-6 \times 10^6$ macrophages

6.500 <u>Collection of Mouse Alveolar Macrophages</u>

6.501 Materials

Animals

Mice 8-12 wk old

Equipment

1-cc TB syringe with 26-gauge needle

Dissecting board(s)

Small scissors (e.g., iris)

Small forceps (e.g., iris)

Laminar flow hood

19- to 21-gauge needles without bevel

3-cc syringe(s)

Petri dish(es)

50-ml tube(s)

Ice bucket

Refrigerated centrifuge 1,000 rpm - 200xg

37°C water bath

Thermometer

Reagents

Nembutal (9 mg pentobarbital sodium/ml)

95% and 70% isopropanol

CMF-HBSS

Gentamicin sulfate (50 μg/ml)

6.502 Preparation for Lavage

1. Set up a water bath at 37°C in a horizontal laminar airflow hood. In addition, place a beaker of 95% ethanol, forceps, scissors, and a Bunsen burner in the hood. Place a sterile beaker in the hood to be used to hold the lavage media.

2. Add gentamicin sulfate (1 cc/500 ml) to prewarmed (37°C) CMF-HBSS in the hood. Pour the media into the prepared sterile beaker and then place it in the water bath in the hood.

3. Place an ice bucket in the hood with the appropriate number of collection vessels, usually one 50-ml centrifuge tube per 3-5 mice. (If the mice were pretreated, one vessel for each treatment group is sufficient).

4. Cut the Luer lock from the tips of 3-cc syringes (one syringe for each mouse), using scissors or scapel. Place the syringes in a sterile Petri dish.

5. Place sterile 20- or 19-gauge needles without bevels (one needle for each mouse) in a sterile Petri dish.

6. Anesthetize the mice with an i.p. injection of 0.3 cc Nembutal (9 mg pentobarbital sodium/ml). In 2-5 min the mice will be anesthetized and can be pinned, 3-5 mice to a dissecting board.

7. Disinfect the surgical field (ventral side) with 70% ethanol. Exsanguinate mice by severing one or both renal arteries in order to minimize postmortem edema and to reduce the amount of blood trapped in the lungs.

8. Remove the skin from the chest by a straight central cut from liver to chin. Pull with both forceps to expose entire chest area. Carefully remove salivary gland, exposing the trachea. Try not to sever the blood vessels on either side of the salivary gland.

9. Open chest cavity from the anterior end of the rib cage, making a straight midline cut down the sternum, exposing the lungs and heart. Do NOT prick or cut lungs or heart. Carefully cut away the rib cage on either side of the lungs, leaving approximately 0.5 cm of the rib cage.

10. The mice can now be placed in the hood and subsequent procedure accomplished aseptically.

6.503 Lavage

1. Remove the membrane from each trachea and make a pinpoint cut in the trachea at the cricoid cartilage.

2. Insert the needles into each trachea. Do not push down beyond the apex of the trachea, because further insertion will result in either puncturing the trachea or entering one of the bronchi (thus only part of the lung would be lavaged).

3. Attach a 3-cc syringe to the hub of each needle containing 2 cc of CMF-HBSS (obtained from prepared beaker). Slowly inject 0.5 cc at a time into each lung until 0.5 cc remains. Withdraw the fluid from the lungs. Expected yield is 1 cc; the rest will re main in the lungs, filling air spaces.

4. Dispense fluid into a 50-ml tube set in ice. Repeat this proce five times for each mouse. The yield should be 1.5-2 cc per lavage step.

   Expected cell yield: 10^5 minimum/mouse; 3×10^5 maximum/mouse.

Notes:

1. The lavage itself is done in an assembly line fashion with 3-5 mice at a time.

2. The syringe and the needle should be kept flat at all times. It is sometimes helpful to place another dissecting board in front of the one the mice are pinned to for the syringes to rest on. If the needle points up or down, it can easily tear the trachea, resulting in loss of macrophages.

6.600   Collagenase Dissociation of Tumors

6.601   Reagents

Methoxy flurane

Ethanol (70%) + iodine solution

HBSS (sterile)

Collagenase solution (sterile) containing:

   HBSS as diluent

   Collagenase, type I, 0.14%

   Deoxyribonuclease (DNAse) I, 0.03%

Trypan blue solution (0.2%)

WBCF diluting fluid: 1% aqueous acetic acid with crystal violet,
   100 mg/liter

Cell culture medium

Freezing medium: see 6.600

6.602   Materials

Dissecting board

Dissecting instruments (sterile)

Petri dishes (sterile)

Trypsinization flasks (sterile)

Stainless steel tissue 80-mesh sieve (sterile)

Magnetic stirring apparatus

Adhesive tape, preferably masking tape

Pasteur pipettes (sterile)

50-ml centrifuge tubes, conical (sterile)

Centrifuge, room temperature, capable of 200-400 X g

Hemacytometer

Light microscope, 100 and 400 magnifications

37°C water bath

6.603   Tumor Excision

1.   Kill mouse by cervical dislocation or anesthetic overdose.

2.   Disinfect mice with iodine solution by total immersion and
     then wash in 70% ethanol.

3.   Immobilize mice on dissecting board.

4.   Disinfect the surgical field with 70% ethanol.

5.   Aseptically excise tumor tissue after removing the adherent
     skin and connective tissue. Avoid (dissect free) the central,
     often necrotic, areas.

6. Rinse tumor tissue in HBSS in a Petri dish to remove serosangui nous fluid; trim necrotic areas, connective tissue, and blood clots.

7. To increase surface area for digestion, mince the tissue with scissors (or crossed scapel blades) into 1- to 2-mm pieces.

6.604 Dissociation

1. Add the minced tumor tissue to the trypsinization flask.

2. Add collagenase-DNAse solution and a magnetic stir bar.

3. Place flask on a magnetic stirrer in a 37°C water bath.

4. Allow to stir at a speed that results in consistent agitation without frothing.

5. After 30 min pour off collagenase-DNAse solution containing single cells.

6. Add fresh 37°C collagenase-DNAse and repeat steps 4-6 a total of three times.

7. After each dissociation, centrifuge the cells and wash once with HBSS. Store cells on ice until all three dissociations are completed.

8. Filter cells through the stainless steel tissue sieve and sus pend in HBSS.

9. Using the hemacytometer, determine the viable cell count by try blue exclusion. (Use only preparations that are $>$ 85% viable.)

6.700 <u>Cryopreservation of Collagenase-Dissociated Cell Suspensions</u>

6.701 Cell Preparation

1. Determine cell concentration, centrifuge, and resuspend to not less than 4×10^7 cells/ml or more than 10×10^7 cells/ml serum free medium (on ice).

2. Prepare freezing medium (2X) (ice cold):

5% Human serum albumin (to prevent the incorporation of FB antigens and allow a tumor challenge with tissue cultur propagated tumor cells)

15% DMSO

80% HBSS

3. Combine cell suspension and freezing medium (equal volumes) for a final concentration of

2.5% human serum albumin

7.5% DMSO

87.5% cell suspension in serum-free medium

4. Apportion 1-2 ml cell suspension to each of several Nunc freezing vials. Store vials on ice.

5. Follow procedure listed in 4.700 to freeze the cells or use a controlled rate freezer.

6.800 <u>Irradiation of Tumor Cells</u>

6.801 Preparation of Cells

1. Wash cells as required by diluting out the DMSO very slowly using HBSS.

2. Centrifuge to remove DMSO.

3. Suspend cells in about 20 ml HBSS.

4. Determine total cell count and volume required for 10^8 cells/ml.

5. Place cells in a beaker of ice for irradiation.

6.900 <u>Cloning by Limiting Dilution in Micro Test II Plates</u>

1. Use an actively growing tumor cell line in mid log phase of culture.

2. Clone cells in conditioned medium (48-hr culture medium from the cells to be cloned). Filter sterilize to remove any tumor cells and mix 50:50 with fresh medium.

3. Harvest tumor cells to produce a single-cell suspension (CMF-HBSS).

4. Count cells and dilute to 3-5 cells/ml in 50:50 conditioned medium.

5. Add 100 µl of cells-medium to each well of a micro test II plate. During the plating period, agitate the cell supension regularly. Feed with 100 µ 50:50 conditioned medium.

6. Add 200 µl of cells-medium to each well of another micro test II plate. Agitate cells regularly.

7. Incubate for 24 hr and identify wells containing a single cell.

8. Incubate until wells, about one in three, develop a partial monolayer.

9. Trypsinize 15 wells and add cells from each well to an individual T-25 culture flask.

Note a: If more than 50% of the cells develop monolayers, too many cells were seeded.

Note b: It is vital that the cells added to each well be in single cell suspension.

Note c: It may be necessary to refeed wells once a week to avoid dehydration of wells.

Note d: It is sometimes possible, because of the formation of multiple colonies in a single well, to determine if a culture started from multiple cells.

6.1000 Preparation of Mononuclear Cells From Blood or the Separation of Viable Cells From a Mixed Cell Population

6.1001 Reagents and Equipment

Blood sample (cell samples)

Hanks' balanced salt solution (HBSS) containing no calcium or magnesium (CMF-HBSS)

Ficoll-Hypaque

Medium

Low speed centrifuge

Sterile 15- or 50-ml tubes

6.1002 Procedure

1. Obtain 15-20 ml blood in a heparinized container.

2. Dilute with 2 volumes of CMF-HBSS.

3. Layer 8 ml of diluted cell suspension over 4 ml of Ficoll-Hypaque in a 15-ml centrifuge tube or 15 ml over 30 ml Ficoll-Hypaque.

4. Centrifuge at room temperature at 850 x g for 20 min. Mononuclear cells or viable cells should form a visible, clean interface between the plasma and Ficoll-Hypaque.

5. Aspirate the plasma and retain the mononuclear cell layer. Place cells in a clean 15-ml centrifuge tube.

6. Fill the tube with CMF-HBSS, mix the cells, then centrifuge at 850 x g for 20 min. Aspirate and discard supernate.

7. Resuspend cells in CMF-HBSS, mix, and centrifuge at 300 x g for 5 min. Aspirate and discard supernate.

8. Resuspend cells with 10 ml of complete medium.

For monocyte depletion:

9. Adjust cell suspension to $1-3 \times 10^6$ cells/ml with RPMI-1640

serum. Add cell suspension to tissue culture flask at a depth of ~ 1 cm. Incubate at 37°C for 60 min in a CO_2 incubator.

10. Decant nonadherent lymphocytes to a clean centrifuge tube. Rinse culture flask gently with 1/10 volume of MEM, adding this liquid to the centrifuge tube. Spin at 300 x g for 5 min. Aspirate and discard supernate.

11. Resuspend cells in complete medium, mix gently, and determine cell viability. Cells should be > 90% viable.

6.1100 Murine Peripherial Blood Lymphocyte

1. Exsanguinate mice by retinal orbital puncture into a heparinized Pasteur pipette.

2. Dilute blood 1:3 into Ca^{++}-Mg^{++}-free HBSS.

3. Layer over 8 ml of Lymphoprep-M in a 15-ml polystyrene tube.

4. Centrifuge at room temperature at 850 x g for 20 min.

5. Aspirate the plasma and retain the mononuclear cell layer (interface). Place cells in a clean 15-ml centrifuge tube.

6. Fill the tube with CMF-HBSS, mix the cells, and then centrifuge at 850 x g for 20 min. Aspirate and discard supernate.

7. Resuspend cells in CMF-HBSS, and centrifuge at 300 x g for 5 min. Aspirate and discard supernate.

8. Resuspend cells from the pellet.

6.1200 Isolation of Pulmonary NK Cells

6.1201 Equipment

1-cc TB syringe with 26-gauge needle

Dissecting board(s)

Small sissors

Small forceps

19- to 22-gauge needles without bevel

Magnetic stirring apparatus

3-cc syringes

Petri dishes

50-ml tubes

Ice bucket

37°C water bath

Thermometer

Refrigerated centrifuge

Scalpels

15-cc sterile tubes

Trypsinization flasks (sterile)

Nembutal (9 mg pentobarbital sodium/ml)

95% and 70% alcohol

Gentamicin sulfate

Collagenase solution (sterile containing) HBSS with 0.14% collagenase and 0.03% DNA

6.1202 Reagents

HBSS containing no calcium or magnesium

Appropriate medium

6.1203 Procedure

1. Anethatize the mice and harvest the alveolar macrophages using a tracheal-bronchial lavage (see 6.4000)

2. Remove the lungs and dissect away the heart, thymic tissue, and external bronchiolar tissue.

3. Mince the pulmonary tissue using crossed scalpel blades to obtain 1-mm^3 fragments.

4. Dissociate the minced tissue with collagenase and DNA (see 6.5

5. Wash the dissociated cells thoroughly and layer onto Lymphoprep-M (6.1000).

6.1300 <u>Isolation of Hepatic NK Cells and Kupffer Cells.</u> (26)

6.1301 Equipment

1-cc TB syringe with 26-gauge needle

Dissecting board

Small sissors

Small forceps

21-gauge butterfly needle

50-gauge stainless steel mech

37°C water bath

Trypsinization flask

Magnetic stirrer

50-cc syringe

Petri dish

50-ml tube

Refrigerated centrifuge

15-ml conial tube

6.1302   Reagents

CMF-HBSS

Medium - 5% FBS

Heparin

95% and 70% alcohol

HBSS containing 0.14% collagenase, 0.03% DNA, and 5% FBS

Gey's solution

Metrizamide

6.1303   Procedure

1. Anesthetize mice. Cut the inferior vena cava to allow rapid exsanguination.

2. Expose the hepatic portal vein and catheterize using a 21-gauge butterfly needle and a 50-cc syringe. Flush the liver with 8-10 ml prewarmed RPMI-1880 containing 5% FBS and heparin. When properly performed, the liver becomes completely blanched.

3. Mince the livers into 1-cm^3 fragments and force the fragments through a stainless steel mesh using a sterile syringe plunger.

4. Wash the cell fragments and dissociate with collagenase (see 6.500) using 10 ml of solution to 1 ml packed cell volume.

5. Wash the cells two times in cold HBSS.

6. Mix the single cell suspension in HBSS with 30% metrizamide in Gey's solution to give a final ratio of 7 parts metrizamide to 5 parts cells in HBSS.

7. Add 5 ml of this mixture to a 15-ml conical centrifuge tube.

8. Overlay the mixture with 1.5 ml HBSS and centrifuge at 1,400 x g for 20 min at 4°C.

9. Carefully remove the nonparenchymal cell layer with a Pasteur pipette and wash the cells two times in complete medium.

6.1400   Isolation of Large Granular Lymphocytes by Percoll Density Gradient Centrifugation (27)

6.1401   Reagents
       Medium
       Percoll
       Sterile distilled water
       Phosphate-buffered saline (10x)

6.1402   Equipment
       Refractometer
       Osmometer
       Centrifuge
       1-, 2-, 5-, and 10-ml pipettes
       15-ml conical test tube

6.1403   Procedure

1. Adjust medium and Percoll to 285 mosmol with sterile distilled water and 10 x phosphate-buffered saline (pH 7.4).

2. Seven different concentrations of Percoll medium are prepared, ranging from 38.6 to 70.1% Percoll, 138.6, 47.5, 52.1, 56.5, 61.1, 65.6, and 70.1%.

4. Make a discontinuous density gradient in the 15-ml conical tubes using seven 1.5-ml steps.

5. After carefully layering the discontinuous gradient, place 5×10^7 lymphocytes in medium on the top of the gradient.

6. Centrifuge the tubes at 550 x g for 30 min at room temperature

7. Collect cells from the seven layers from the discontinuous gradient with a Pasteur pipette and wash once in medium.

7.000   TECHNIQUES USED IN MECHANISM STUDIES

7.100   <u>Preparation and Use of Nylon Wool Columns for T-Cell Enrichment</u> (28

7.101   Reagents
       Distilled water (glass distilled)
       EDTA
       RPMI-1640 medium (5% ΔFBS) + HEPES
       Sodium bicarbonate

7.102   Materials
       Aluminum foil
       Autoclave bags

Column stand

Disposable gloves

50-ml conical-bottom centrifuge tubes

1-, 5-, and 10-ml pipettes

4-liter glass beaker

Incubator (37°C with 5% CO_2)

Large tray covered with absorbent paper

Nylon wool (Fenwall Laboratories)

Stainless steel basket or funnel

10- and 30-cc syringes

3-way stopcocks

22-gauge needles

37°C water bath

7.103 Procedure

7.103a Washing and Drying of Nylon Wool

1. When handling nylon wool, wear disposable latex gloves that have been rinsed free of powder with distilled water. Remove nylon wool from one or two bulk packages (35 g each) and place in a glass beaker with 4 liters of freshly boiled distilled water containing 0.2% sodium bicarbonate (2 g/liter) and 0.2% EDTA (2 g/liter). Soak overnight at 37°C.

2. Squeeze out excess water and place nylon wool in a 4-liter glass beaker of distilled water. Cover the beaker with aluminum foil and boil for approximately 10 min.

3. Allow the water and nylon wool to cool to room temperature. Decant water and drain the nylon wool in a stainless steel basket or funnel.

4. Repeat the washing procedure (steps 1-3) a total of six times in freshly distilled water each time.

5. Squeeze out excess water and spread the wet nylon wool on a tray covered with absorbent paper (filter paper). Dry nylon wool in a laminar flow hood for 2-3 days. Store in a covered glass container.

7.103b Packing of Nylon Wool Columns (28, 29)

1. Determine the total number of cells to be passed through a column (yields are 50%). Use the information from the following table to determine the size of syringe and the weight of nylon required.

No. of cells	Capacity of syringe	Nylon wool/syringe
1×10^8	10 ml	0.6 gm
3×10^8	30 ml	1.8 gm
4×10^8	30 ml	2.4 gm

2. Weigh nylon wool. Tease apart, separating the strands until the piece is loosely connected yet free of tangles and knots. Loosely fold nylon wool so that it will fit the diameter of the syringe and pack the syringe.

3. For sterile work, pack individual syringes into autoclaving bags and autoclave at 121°C for 15 min. Autoclave plungers separately if they are to be used alone.

7.103c Cell Separation

1. Warm RPMI-1640 (5% ΔFBS) + HEPES to 37°C in a water bath.

2. In a laminar airflow hood, mount syringe containing sterile nylon wool in a column stand and attach the 3-way stopcock and a capped 22-gauge needle to the syringe. Remove the needle cap, open the stopcock, and thoroughly rinse the nylon wool with 50-100 ml of prewarmed medium. Close the stopcock, add medium to cover the nylon wool, and free column of air bubbles by agitation with a pipette.

3. Gently insert the syringe plunger and replace needle cap. Incubate the column at 37°C for 1 hr.

4. While the column is incubating, prepare the cell suspension and adjust the concentration to approximately 5×10^7 cells/ml in prewarmed medium.

5. Just before adding the cell suspension, rinse the wool with 5-10 ml of prewarmed medium, let column run dry, and close stopcock. Add the appropriate number of cells (refer to the table under preparation of columns), and allow cells to penetrate the column by opening the stopcock. Add an additional 0.5 ml of medium, gently insert the syringe plunger, close the stopcock, and replace the needle cap. Maintain the column at 37°C for 45 min.

6. Collect nonadherent cells into a 50-ml centrifuge tube by washing the 10- to 12-ml column with 20 ml of prewarmed medium and the 35-ml column with 60 ml of medium. Elute at about 1 drop/sec. Centrifuge cells (1,200 rpm for 6 min) and resuspend in the appropriate assay medium.

Notes:

1. When using RPMI-1640 medium, 25 mM HEPES must be added to prevent the medium from becoming alkaline.

2. To recover adherent cells from the column, add cold saline (0.85% NaCl) to the column and forcibly push fluid out with the plunger.

3. It is possible to recycle nylon wool. After use, rinse the nylon in saline and then place in 0.1 M HCl at least overnight. Repeat washing procedures as before. Some lots may work at least as well, if not better, after recycling.

4. The loss of Fc-receptor-positive T cells on nylon wool is variable. The loss is increased by tightly packing the nylon but is rarely complete; it may vary with the batch.

5. In general, T cells pass through nylon wool, whereas B cells and macrophages are retained. However, some functional subpopulations of T cells may adhere to the columns. Functional subpopulations of T cells reported to pass through the columns include primed and unprimed antigen-specific helper cells, T cells that are the precursors of cytotoxic effectors, and T cells that proliferate in response to both alloantigens and soluble antigens.

6. The passage of cells through a nylon wool column is an effective means of obtaining a population enriched with T cells. B cells, plasma cells, and some accessory cells preferentially adhere to the nylon wool, whereas many T cells (and some null cells) pass through the column. Yields are often low, in the range of 15%-25%. Most investigators have found that the T cells present in the effluent are representative of all T-cell subpopulations. However, other studies suggest that T-cell subpopulations are selectively retained on nylon wool. Such selective retention may, if confirmed, be due to variations in nylon wool lots, the degree to which the column is packed, and/or the preparative washing procedures used.

7.200 Preparation of Liposomes: Multilamillar Vesicles (MLV) (30,31)

7.201 Equipment

Glass tubes with teflon-lined cap

Centrifuge with 55-34 head

Desiccator jar

Vacuum punp

Rotary, evaporator vacuum

Waterbath at 36°C

Vortex with tube stand

Nucleopore filter 0.5-mm

Glass pipettes and pipette aid

7.202 Reagents

Argon or nitrogen

Phosphotidylcholine

Phosphatidylserine

HBSS

Chloroform

Methanol

7.203 Preparatory Steps

7.203a Washing of Glassware

1. Scrub with a small amount of dilute phosphate free detergent solution.

2. Rinse with distilled water. Autoclave. Store at room temperature.

3. Before use, rinse with absolute ethanol or methanol to remove residual moisture.

4. Rinse with chloroform twice and allow to dry.

7.203b Preparation of Lipid

1. Remove chromatographically pure preparations of lipid, dissolved in chloroform from storage at -70°C.

2. Prepare stock solution of lipids (e.g., 10 μmol lipid/ml chloroform) according to the following table. (Store at -20°C.

Phospholipid	Formula weight	Amt. lipid/ml $CHCl_3$ to yield 10 $\mu mol/ml$
Phosphatidylcholine (PC) (Egg lecithin)	785	7.85 μg
Phosphatidylserine (PS)	811	8.11 μg

3. Hold all solutions powders on ice. Return to -70°C or -20°C as appropriate immediately.

4. Store in tubes with a Teflon-lined cap. It is best to store in tubes filled to the top (to prevent oxidation) or purged with argon or nitrogen.

5. Solubilize MTP-PE in 20% methanol and 80% chloroform immediately before use and add to chloroform-soluble PC and PS, i.e., 70 $\mu mole$ PC, 30 $\mu mole$ PS, and 40 $\mu mole$ MTP-PE.

6. Using a pipette and propipette (or equivalent pipetting device), transfer 10-100 $\mu mole$ lipid to a round-bottomed, glass, screw-capped tube (50 ml).

7. Never use grease in any joints of the rotary vacuum vaporator.

8. Evaporate the lipid solution to dryness by placing the tube onto the rotary vacuum evaporator.

Note: Large volumes (e.g., >10 ml) should be chilled in an ice bath to prevent boiling when vacuum is applied.

9. Turn the vacuum pump on.

10. Turn the rotary motor on (indicator set at 4-6) and align the tube so that it rotates smoothly.

11. Lower the tube into the waterbath (approximately 36°C).

12. Remove the chloroform by evaporation until the lipid forms a dry film or shell on the inner surface of the tube (requires 1-1.5 min/ml $CHCl_3$).

13. After formation of lipid film, raise the tube out of the waterbath.

14. Turn the rotary motor off.

15. Turn the vacuum pump off and grasp the tube.

16. Flush the tube with argon and tightly cap the tube in order to maintain anaerobiosis. Rapidly transfer to a desiccator jar.

17. Complete the drying process by placing the lipid films in a desiccator jar connected to a high-vacuum pump for a minimum of 60 min.

18. Exercise caution in opening the jar to prevent dust from entering the tubes.

19. These "shells" can be stored at -70°C.

7.204   Preparation of Liposomes

1. Add aqueous immunostimulant solutions (1-10 ml, usually 1 ml for each milliliter of stock lipid solution) to the tubes to hydrate the dried films.

2. Hydration of the lipid in CMF-HBSS should take place for 5-10 min at 37°C with gentle rotation.

3. Vortex the lipid solution for 10 min at room temperature (argon atmosphere). MLV are formed when the lipid is dispersed in the aqueous phase during vortexing.

4. Transfer the preparation to high-speed plastic centrifuge tubes for centrifugation. Fill the tube with CMF-HBSS and centrifuge at 20,000 x g (Sorvall RC2-B centrifuge, SS-34 head, 17,500 rpm for 15 to 20 min. Decant the supernatant, being careful not to disturb the pellet. Repeat the washing one time.

Note: Liposomes containing only lipophilic MTP-PE as immunostimulant do not require centrifugation. In this case, the lipophilic MDP is added in CHCl₃ to the PS and PC before shell formation

5. Suspend the pelleted liposomes to an appropriate lipid concentration in serum-free culture medium or physiological saline and store at 5°C.

Notes:

1. Since the MLV vary in size (0.1-100 μm), extrusion through a nucleopore filter (e.g., polycarbonate membrane with 0.5-μm pore size) will produce MLV of a more uniform size.

2. Liposomes containing lipophilic MDP are stable. Sterile preparations may be stored at room temperature for extended periods of time. However, following storage for greater than 1 hr, the MLV must be revortexed and extracted through a filter.

3. MLV containing hydrophilic BRM must be used within 1 hr of preparation to avoid leakage.

4. Aqueous material entrapped in MLV is very unstable, and the material diffuses out rapidly. However, such MLV preparations may be stored after vortexing in the original concentration of aqueous material to achieve equilibrium.

5. PS is very unstable and decomposes, with a half-life of 30 days. Thus, fresh PS must be used; it should be ordered monthly.

6. Levels of MLV incorporating MTP-PE

   In vitro: 500 nmoles lipid/ml

   In vivo: murine - 5 μmole lipid in 0.2 ml/mouse

   : rat - 50 μmole lipid in 0.5 ml/rat

7.500 Determination of Cl⁻ Content of Drinking Water

7.501 Reagents and Materials

Water sample

Sodium hypochloride (NaOCl)

UV spectrophotometer

7.502 Assay of Cl⁻ Content

1. Prepare a standard solution of 0.01% (100 ppm) NaOCl in deionized water.

2. Construct a standard curve with the standard solution by preparing a serial dilution in deionized water (linear curve).

3. Read the OD of the standards at 295 μm. (Be sure to warm UV lamp prior to reading OD.)

4. Plot data to form the standard curve.

5. Read unknown at 295 μm and determine ppm against the standard curve.

Note: NaOCl is not stable, and available chlorine may decay with time.

8.000 ALLOGENEIC MIXED LYMPHOCYTE REACTION (MLR) ASSAY (32-34)

8.100 Reagents

HBSS

Scintillation fluid

Trypan blue dye

[³H]Thymidine (stock solution, 50 μCi/ml)

EHAA + 0.5% NMS

8.200   Materials

96-well microtiter plates (Costar-flat bottom)

50-ml conical-bottom centrifuge tubes

12 x 75-mm RTU tubes

1-, 5-, 10-ml Pasteur pipettes

Microdoser with sterile tips

Hemacytometer

Compound research microscope

Humidified, 5% CO_2 incubator

Scintillation vials

24-well cell harvestor

Beta counter

37°C water bath

Refrigerated centrifuge (Beckman TJ-6)

8.300   <u>Procedure</u>

1. Remove spleens from mice (C57BL/6 and C3H) and prepare a single cell suspension (see section 6.100).

2. Wash cells 1X in HBSS and resuspend in a conical-bottom tube at 10^7 cells/ml.

3. Irradiate an aliquot of each spleen cell concentration (2,000 R

4. Count cells and adjust to a concentration of 7.5 x 10^5 cells/ml (irradiated stimulator (S) cells) or 1 x 10^7 cells/ml (non-irradiated responder (R) cells). Suspend cells at this concentration in EHAA + 0.5% NMS.

5. Remove five 2.0-ml aliquots from each of the responder cell suspensions (1 x 10^7 cells/ml) and mix with 2.0 ml of medium containing a different dose of BRM. Store spleen cells on ice until plated.

8.400   <u>Plating</u>

The groups listed below are routinely plated for each MLR assay in quadruplicate wells on two separate plates (plates I and II). The various cells and medium are plated in 0.1-ml volumes, respectively so that the final volume per well is 0.2 ml. Thymosin fraction 5 serves as the positive control.

96-WELL MICROTITER PLATE (FLAT BOTTOM)

	C3H R only Wells (1-4)	C3H R_S +C3H^S Wells (5-8)	C3H R_S +C57^S Wells (9-12)
ROW			
A	Medium		
B	100 µg/ml Thymosin F-5		
C	BRM Dose #1		
D	Dose #2		
E	Dose #3		
F	Dose #4		
G	Dose #5		

1. Lightly vortex cells and transfer responder cells (nonirra-diated cells) in 100 µl of medium or medium with the BRM to the appropriate wells of a 96-well microtiter plate (four wells/group). Use 96-well plates with tight lids.
2. Remove any moisture on the lids with a sterile Pasteur pipette.
3. Transfer the appropriate stimulator cell population to the wells in a 100-µl aliquot (lightly vortex suspensions first).
4. Remove any moisture on the lids with a sterile Pasteur pipette.
5. Incubate at 37°C in a high humidity incubator.
6. On day 3 of incubation, add 1 µCi of [^{3}H]thymidine (0.02 ml volume) to the wells of plate I, and on day 4 add 1 µCi of [^{3}H]thymidine to the wells of plate II. Harvest the plates via a 24-well cell harvester 18-20 hr after the addition of the label.
7. Transfer the filter paper discs from the cell harvester to vials containing 1.0 ml of scintillation fluid and determine cpm on a beta counter.

8.500 Representation of Data

Express the data as average cpm ± the standard error for each group, or calculate the stimulation index (SI) and the relative proliferation index (RPI):

$$SI = \frac{\text{cpm experimental allogeneic culture - cpm control responder culture}}{\text{cpm control responder culture}}$$

$$RPI = \frac{\text{cpm experimental allogeneic culture - cpm control responder culture}}{\text{cpm control allogeneic culture - cpm control responder culture}}$$

9.000   ALLOGENEIC MIXED LYMPHOCYTE TUMOR REACTION - CELL-MEDIATED
           CYTOTOXICITY (MLTR-CMC) (35-40)

9.100   <u>Reagents</u>

HBSS

EHAA + 0.5% NMS

Triton X-100 (1% solution in water)

Trypan blue

Sodium [51]chromate (1 mCi/ml)

Pooled NMS

9.200   <u>Materials</u>

T-25 flasks

96-well microtiter plates (Linbro-U bottom)

15-ml conical-bottom centrifuge tubes

50-ml conical-bottom centrifuge tubes

12 x 75-mm glass tubes

1-, 5-, 10-ml pipettes; Pasteur pipettes

Microdoser - sterile tips

Hemacytometer

Compound research microscope

Humidified, 5% CO_2 incubator

Titertek Supernatant Collection System

Gamma counter

Refrigerated centrifuge (Beckman TJ-6)

37°C water bath

9.300   <u>Treatment of P815 Cells</u>

1. Irradiate the P815 cells (5,000 R).

2. Perform a cell count and adjust the concentration of P815
cells to 8×10^4/ml (for Falcon T-25 flask) or 1×10^5/ml
(for Corning T-25 flask) in EHAA + 0.5% NMS. A total of 7
ml is required for five doses of a BRM and the necessary
controls. Store cells on ice until used.

9.400   Preparation of MLTR-CMC Spleen Cells

1. Remove the spleens from the appropriate mice (C3H) and prepare a single-cell suspension as described in section 6.100.

2. Perform a viable cell count using trypan blue stain and adjust the spleen cell concentration to 2.5×10^7/ml (for
   Falcon T-25 flask) or 3×10^7/ml (for Corning T-25 flask)
   in EHAA + 0.5% NMS. A total of 14 ml is required for five
   doses of a BRM and the necessary controls.

9.500   Incubation of MLTR-CMC

1. The groups listed below are routinely incubated together for
   each MLTR-CMC assay in a T-25 flask. The responder-to-stimulator ratio is usually 300:1. When using the Falcon T-25
   plastic flask, the cell numbers to be added are 2.5×10^7
   viable responder C_3H spleen lymphocytes and 8×10^4 viable
   stimulator x-irradiated P815 tumor cells. When using the
   Corning T-25 flask, the ratio of responder-to-stimulator
   cells is the same, but as the resting surface differs from
   that of the Falcon flask, the cell numbers are adjusted to
   3×10^7 responders and 1×10^5 stimulators. Final volume
   per flask is 20 ml. Each BRM dose is prepared at 2X concentration in EHAA 0.5% NMS; 20 ml is needed per dose. Thymosin
   F5 serves as the positive control.

Group	Medium	BRM	Responder	Stimulator
1	19 ml	None	1 ml	None
2	9 ml	10 ml dose 1 (2X)	1 ml	None
3	9 ml	10 ml dose 2 (2X)	1 ml	None
4	9 ml	10 ml dose 3 (2X)	1 ml	None
5	9 ml	10 ml dose 4 (2X)	1 ml	None
6	9 ml	10 ml dose 5 (2X)	1 ml	None
7	9 ml	10 ml Thymosin Fraction 5 (200 µg/ml = 2X)	1 ml	None
8	18 ml	None	1 ml	1 ml
9	8 ml	10 ml dose 1 (2X)	1 ml	1 ml
10	8 ml	10 ml dose 2 (2X)	1 ml	1 ml
11	8 ml	10 ml dose 3 (2X)	1 ml	1 ml
12	8 ml	10 ml dose 4 (2X)	1 ml	1 ml
13	8 ml	10 ml dose 5 (2X)	1 ml	1 ml
14	8 ml	10 ml Thymosin Fraction 5 (200 µg/ml = 2X)	1 ml	1 ml

2. Incubate the flasks at 37°C in a humidified, 5% CO_2 incubator for a total of 5 days.

3. On day 5 of incubation, collect the cells from the T-25 flasks for each experimental group. Prepare the lymphocytes for use in a 4-hr ^{51}Cr-release cytotoxicity assay by washing the cells 1X in RPMI (5% FBS). Perform a total and viable cell count in trypan blue stain and adjust the viable cells to 5×10^6/ml, 2.5×10^6/ml, 1.2×10^6/ml, and 6×10^5/ml, respectively, in supplemented RPMI-1640 + 5% FBS.

4. If the viability of the cells is poor, it may be necessary to resuspend a pellet of spleen cells in 10 ml of FBS. Let the suspension for 30 to 60 min and remove the viable, non-clumped spleen cells.

9.600 Cytotoxicity Testing of MLTR-CMC (4-hr ^{51}Cr-Release Assay)

9.601 ^{51}Cr-Labeling of P815 Target Cells (See 4.603)

9.602 Plating of MLTR-CMC 4-hr ^{51}Cr-Release Assay

The following 4-hr ^{51}Cr-release assay is carried out on day 5 of the MLTR-CMC assay.

1. Plate all dilutions of a given MLTR spleen cell preparation in triplicate in a volume of 0.1 ml in a 96-well microtiter plate (Linbro-U Bottom). Routinely plate effector/target ratios of 50:1, 25:1, 12:1, and 6:1 (5×10^5, 2.5×10^5, 1.25×10^5, and 6×10^4 lymphocytes, respectively).

2. If desired, unlabeled tumor cells can be used as negative specificity control.

3. To each well add 10^4 ^{51}Cr-labeled P815 cells in a volume of 0.1 ml.

4. Be sure to plate ^{51}Cr-labeled P815 cells for determination of autologous and maximum release. Autologous release is determined by incubating 0.1 ml of labeled cells (10^4) with 0.1 ml of nonlabeled P815 cells (5×10^5, 2.5×10^5, 1.25×10^5, and 6×10^4) respectively. Maximum release is determined by incubating 0.1 ml of Triton X-100 with 0.1 ml of labeled P815 cells (10^4).

5. Centrifuge plates at 800 rpm for 5 min.

6. Incubate plates at 37°C in a humidified, 5% CO_2 incubator for 4 hr.

7. Centrifuge plates at 800 rpm for 5 min.
8. Collect radioactive supernatant fluids using the Titertek Supernatant Collection System.
9. Transfer radioactive plugs from plastic tubes to 12 x 75 mm glass tubes and place in gamma counter.

9.700 Calculation of Percent Cytotoxicity (31-36)

$$\frac{cpm\ (released\ experimental) - cpm\ (released\ spontaneously)}{cpm\ (total\ triton\ x\ released) - cpm\ (released\ spontaneously)} \times 100$$

10.000 SUPPRESSOR CELL-HELPER CELL ASSAYS (41)

To demonstrate that a decreased (or increased) response in an immunological assay is due to an active regulation by a suppressor (or helper) cell population, it is necessary to transfer that population to another unstimulated cell population. Therefore, the sensitized cells are added to fresh spleen cells, capable of generating a normal response, and their effector cell function is examined following co-culture with or without stimulator cells. This form of assay provides a functional assessment of the ability of a putative suppressor cell or helper cell to regulate a normal response.

10.100 Reagents

HBSS
EHAA + 0.5% NMS
Triton X-100 (1% solution in water)
Trypan blue
Sodium ^{51}chromate (1 mCi/ml)
Pooled NMS

10.200 Materials

T-25 flasks
96-well microtiter plates (Linbro-U bottom)
15-ml conical-bottom centrifuge tubes
50-ml conical-bottom centrifuge tubes
12 x 75-RTU tubes
1-, 5-, 10-ml pipettes; Pasteur pipettes
Microdoser - sterile tips
Hemacytometer

Compound research microscope

Humidified, 5% CO_2 incubator

Titertek Supernatant Collection System

Gamma counter

Refrigerated centrifuge (Beckman TJ-6)

37°C water bath

10.300 Preparation of a Secondary MLTR Culture

1. On day 5 of the incubation of the primary MLTR (see 9.000), collect the cells from the T-25 flasks for each experimental group. Prepare the lymphocytes for addition to the second MLTR by washing once in EHAA.

2. Perform a total and viable cell count in trypan blue.

3. The cell populations (from the primary 5 day cultures) are added in graded numbers to a second MLTR culture.

4. The putative regulatory cells are added at ratios of 0:1, 0.1:1, 1:1, and 2:1 to normal spleen cells in a second MLTR co-cultur

5. The total number of spleen cells added per flask is held constant at 2.5×10^7 cells/flask:

a) regulator cells 0×10 : fresh cell 2.5×10^7

b) " " 2.5×10^6 : " " 2.2×10^7

c) " " 1.25×10^7: " " 1.25×10^7

d) " " 1.67×10^7: " " 0.83×10^7

6. Suppressor cell assays are initiated at a near optimal stimulator: responder (S:R) cell ratios, i.e., 1:50 with 2×10^6 P815 stimulator cells and 2.5×10^7 responder cells. In contrast, helper cell assays are initiated at a very suboptimal stimulator-to-responder cell ratio, i.e., 1:700 with 3.5×10^4 P815 stimulator cells and 2.5×10^7 responder cells.

7. The effector cells are removed, 5 days later, from the seconda MLTR assay and their activity is established in a 4-hr ^{51}Cr-release cytotoxicity assay.

11.000 MEMBRANE PHENOTYPE OF REGULATORY OR EFFECTOR CELLS (41-42)

11.100 Reagents

HBSS

Anti-Thy 1.2 antiserum

Anti-asialo GM1 antiserum

Anti-Lyt 1.2 antiserum
Anti-Lyt 2.2 antiserum
Rabbit complement
Trypan blue
CMEM - 5% FBS
Normal mouse serum (NMS)
HEPES

11.200 Materials

Sterile 12 x 75 glass tubes
1-, 5-, 10-ml pipettes
Micropipette, sterile tips
Hemacytometer
Compound research microscope
Refrigerated centrifuge
37°C water bath

11.300 Antibody Treatment

1. Harvest effector cells from the primary MLTR assay, wash once in medium, and add equal aliquots of cells to each of three tubes per group.

2. Pellet cells, 1,200 rpm for 10 min. Aspirate medium.

3. To tube A (complement control) add 200 µl HBSS, 10 mM HEPES, and 0.5% NMS.
    To tube B add antiserum in 10 mM HEPES and 0.5% NMS.

4. Resuspend and incubate for 60 min at 37°C in a water bath. Shake tubes occasionally.

5. Add to all tubes 100 µl of rabbit complement previously determined to lack independent cytotoxicity.

6. Incubate for 30 min at 37°C in a water bath.

7. Wash cells twice using RPMI-1640.

8. Resuspend cells in 1.2 ml RPMI-1640/5% FBS to be used directly as effector cells in CMC assays (see 9.000) or resuspend the cells at the desired number in EHAA/0.5 NMS to be used as regulator cells in a secondary MLTR (see 10.000).

12.000 CELL-MEDIATED CYTOTOXICITY ASSAY (CTL) (41)

12.100 Reagents

CMEM + 5% and 10% FBS

CMEM + 5% and 10% FBS (methionine free)

Triton X-100 (1% solution in distilled H_2O)

Trypan blue (0.2%)

[^{75}Se]Methionine

CMF-HBSS

1X Trypsin-EDTA

Gentamicin (50 µg/ml)

Collagenase solution (Refer to 8.500)

12.200 Materials

T-75 tissue culture flasks

Costar 96-well microtiter plates

Pipettman P-200

50 ml conical-bottom centrifuge tube

12 x 75-mm glass tubes

1-, 2-, 5-, and 10-ml pipettes

Pasteur pipettes

Microdoser and sterile tips

Hemacytometer

Compound research microscope

Gamma counter

Refrigerated centrifuge

Humidified, 5% CO_2 incubator

27-gauge hypodermic needles

1-cc syringes

12.300 Immunization

1. On day -15, shave mice (three per group) and immunize at five different intradermal sites with a total of 5×10^6 x-irradiat (10,000 R) fresh collagenase dissociated tumor cells. (Refer to 8.500 for Collagenase Dissociation of Tumors.) Use a 1-cc syringe with a 27-gauge needle for i.d. immunization.

2. Give the mice injections at the five sites with 10^6 cells per site at 0.05 ml admixed with either CMF-HBSS (control)

or the BRM in question (atleast three different doses).

3. A negative control must be included (mice given injections of HBSS alone).

4. On day -5, give the mice injections at two sites as in step 2 with 10^6 cells/ site.

12.400 Preparation of Target Cells

1. Use tumor cells in mid log phase of growth cultured in CMEM + 5% FBS, e.g., cells that have been split 24 hr prior to labelling.

2. Wash the cells once with 4 ml of warmed 37°C trypsin-EDTA.

3. Immediately add 0.7 ml 1X trypsin-EDTA to the T-75 flask.

4. When cells begin to detach, agitate flask.

5. Dilute trypsin with 10-ml CMF-HBSS.

6. Pipette cells into a 50-ml centrifuge tube.

7. Add CMF-HBSS to 50-ml volume.

8. Centrifuge cells at 1,200 rpm for 6 min.

9. Remove supernatant fluids.

10. Resuspend cells in CMF-HBSS at 130,000 cells/ml. This will produce 10,000 cells/well by 24 hr after plating.

11. Add target cells (50 µl) to the appropriate wells of a 96-well plate using the following pattern:

```
Row No.      1   2   3   4   5   6   7   8   9   10   11   12
(Do step 11  ↓   ↑   ↓   ↑   ↓   ↑   ↓   ↑   ↓   ↑    ↓    ↑
first and    ↓   1   ↓   1   ↓   1   ↓   1   ↓   1    ↓    1
step 12 last) 1  8   9   2   7   10  3   6   11  4    5    12
```

This grid ensures the even distribution of aliquoting errors. Frequent light vortexing is required (with cap on tube).

12. Add 50 µl of 50% CMEM and 50% methionine-free medium + 10% FBS.

13. Allow cells to attach for 4 hr at 37°C.

14. Add 0.5 µCi [^{75}Se]methionine to each well in a 100-µl volume in methionine-free CMEM + 5% FBS.

15. Incubate for 16-20 hr.

12.500   Assay (Day 0)

1. Harvest spleens from mice of each of the treatment groups (effectors). Prepare a single cell suspension (Refer to 8.103).

2. Adjust the concentration of the effector groups to 2 x 10^7/ml and place into 5-ml sterile culture tubes in a volume of 1.2 r

3. Aspirate medium from the targets.

4. Wash the targets 4X; use the multiple suction device and warme CMEM + 5% FBS. After final wash, add 100 μl CMEM + 5% FBS to each well.

5. Add effector cells to wells in 100 μl. Routinely plate effector-to-target ratios of 200:1, 100:1, 50:1, and 25:1 (2 x 10^6, 1 x 10^6, 5 x 10^5, and 2.5 x 10^5 lymphocytes/well, respectively).

6. Centrifuge plates at 800 rpm for 5 min.

7. Incubate for 16-18 hr at 37°C in a humidified, 5% CO_2 atmosphe

8. Centrifuge plates for 5 min at 800 rpm.

9. Collect radioactive supernatant fluids in a volume of 100 μl using a pipette. Be careful not to disturb the monolayer of cells. For the Triton X released wells, pipette up and down and harvest 200-μl samples/well.

10. Include autologous release controls or thymocytes and spontaneous release and total release, Triton X.

11. Calculate cytotoxicity using the following equation:

$$\% \text{ cytotoxicity} = \frac{\text{cpm (effector cell released)} - \text{cpm (spontaneo}}{\text{triton x released cpm} - \text{spontaneous release cp}}$$

13.000   NK CELL ASSAY (42-46)

13.100   In Vitro Incubation of Spleen Cells With NK Activation

13.101   Reagents

HBSS

HBSS + 5% ΔFBS

RPMI-1640 medium + 5% ΔFBS + gentamicin

Trypan blue

13.102   Materials

24-well cluster plates (Costar)

50-ml conical-bottom centrifuge tubes

12 x 75 glass tubes

1-, 5-, 10-ml pipettes

Microdoser with sterile tips

Hemacytometer

Compound research microscope

Humidified, 5% CO_2 incubator

Refrigerated centrifuge

13.103   Preparation of Spleen Cells

1.   Remove spleens from 21-day-old weanling mice and prepare single-cell suspensions as described in section 6.100.

2.   Determine the number of viable cells by staining with trypan blue, and adjust the spleen cells to a concentration of 5×10^6/ml in RPMI-1640 medium.   Store on ice until plated.

13.104   Incubation of Spleen Cells With Potential NK Activators

1.   The groups listed below are routinely set up in four wells of a 24-well cluster plate.   Plate 5×10^6 viable lymphocytes in a volume of 1.0 ml of medium.   Five different doses of a medium containing BRM or medium alone are added to four wells of lymphocytes in a volume of 1.0 ml of medium either 24 hr or 2 hr before assessing the NK activity of the cultured lymphocytes.   The NK activity is determined by a 4-hr ^{51}Cr-labeled YAC-1 cell assay.

Poly IC serves as the positive control.

Spleen cells + medium

Spleen cells + poly I:C (5 µg/ml)

Spleen cells + BRM medium (dose #1)

Spleen cells + BRM medium (dose #2)

Spleen cells + BRM medium (dose #3)

Spleen cells + BRM medium (dose #4)

Spleen cells + BRM medium (dose #5)

2.   Incubate the plates for 24 hr at 37°C in a humidified incubator with a 5% CO_2 atmosphere.

3. Collect the cells from the four wells of each experimental group
    After the initial removal of cells and medium from each well, wai
    each well 2X with 1-2 ml of HBSS and pool respective washings.
    Prepare the lymphocytes for use in a 4-hr Cr-release cytotoxicit
    assay by washing them once in HBSS + 5% FBS. Perform a total
    and viable cell count in trypan blue stain and adjust the viable
    cells to concentrations of 5 x 10^6/ml, 2.5 x 10^6/ml, 1.2 x 10^6/m
    and 6 x 10^5/ml, respectively, in RPMI-1640 + 5% ΔFBS.

13.200 NK Cell Assay: ^{51}Cr Release

13.201 Reagents

RPMI-1640 medium

RPMI-1640 medium + 5% ΔFBS

10X HBSS

Trypan blue

Triton X-100 (1% solution in water)

Sterile distilled water

Sodium ^{51}chromate (1 mCi/ml)

13.202 Materials

96-well microtiter plates (Linbro-U bottom)

15-ml conical-bottom centrifuge tubes

50-ml conical-bottom centrifuge tubes

12 x 75-mm glass tubes

1-, 5-, 10-ml pipettes

Microdoser with sterile tips

Hemacytometer

Compound research microscope

Humidified, 5% CO_2 incubator

Titertek Supernatant Collection System

Gamma counter

Refrigerated centrifuge

13.203 ^{51}Cr Labeling of YAC-1 Target Cells (See 4.603)

13.300 Preparation of In Vivo Activated NK Spleen Cells

1. On day -3 (72 hr pretest), inject mice i.v. with HBSS (0.2 ml)
    as control or with HBSS containing one of five different
    dilutions of a BRM. Poly I:C serves as the positive control.

2. On day -1 (24 hr pretest), inject HBSS i.v. (0.2 ml) or HBSS containing one of five different BRM dilutions as well as poly I:C as the positive control.

3. Use 21-day-old C3H mice weaned 72 hr pretest.

4. On day 0, remove spleens and use in the NK cell assay.

5. Remove spleens from the mice and prepare a single-cell suspension as described under section 6.100. Collect spleen cells in serum-free RPMI-1640 medium.

6. Centrifuge spleen cells at 1,200 rpm for at least 6 min.

7. To lyse erythrocytes, resuspend spleen cells pellet into 9 ml of sterile distilled water (3-5 sec). Vortex. Immediately add 1 ml of sterile 10X HBSS. Vortex.

8. Remove cell debris by passing cell suspension through a nylon sieve.

9. Centrifuge spleen cells at 1,200 rpm for at least 6 min. Wash spleen cells in RPMI-1640 medium and resuspend in RPMI-1640 + 5% ΔFBS medium.

10. Perform a cell count and adjust the spleen cells to 5×10^6 viable cells/ml. Store cells on ice until plated.

13.301 Set Up a Short-Term ^{51}Cr-Release Assay

1. Plate all dilutions of a given spleen cell preparation in triplicate in a volume of 0.1 ml in a 96-well microtiter plate (Linbro-U Bottom). Routinely plate effector/target ratios of 50:1, 25:1, 12:1, and 6:1 (5×10^5, 2.5×10^5, 1.25×10^5, and 6×10^4 lymphocytes, respectively).

2. To each well add 10^4 ^{51}Cr-labeled YAC-1 cells in a volume of 0.1 ml.

3. Be sure to plate labeled YAC-1 cells for determination of autologous, spontaneous, and maximum release. Autologous release is determined by incubating 0.1 ml of labeled YAC-1 cells (10^4) with 0.1 ml of nonlabeled YAC-1 cells (5×10^5, 2.5×10^5, 1.25×10^5, and 6×10^4, respectively). Maximum release is determined by incubating 0.1 ml of Triton X-100 with 0.1 ml of labeled YAC-1 cells (10^4).

4. Centrifuge plates at 800 rpm for 5 min.

5. Incubate plates for 4 hr at 37°C in a humidified incubator with 5% CO_2 atmosphere.
6. Centrifuge plates for 5 min at 800 rpm.
7. Collect radioactive supernatant fluids with the use of the Titertek Supernatant Collection System.
8. Transfer radioactive plugs in plastic tubes to 12 x 75-mm glass tubes and place in gamma counter.

13.302 Calculation of Percent Cytotoxicity

$$\frac{\text{cpm released from experimental group} \quad \text{cpm released from autologous control}}{\text{total cpm Triton X released}} \text{ X } 100$$

13.400 NK Cell Assay: Long-Term-[3H]Proline (45)

13.401 Reagents

Supplemented CMEM + 5% ΔFBS

Supplemented CMEM (without nonessential amino acids)

Phosphate-buffered saline (PBS)

10X HBSS

1% Triton X

Scintillation fluid

[3H]proline (20-40 Ci/mmol)

13.402 Materials

96-well microtiter plates (Costar - flat bottom)

50-ml conical-bottom centrifuge tubes

12 x 75-mm glass tubes

1-, 5-, 10-ml pipettes; Pasteur pipettes

Microdoser-sterile tips

Hemacytometer

Compound research microscope

Humidified, 5% CO_2 incubator

Scintillation vials

Beta counter

Refrigerated centrifuge

13.403 [^{3}H]Proline Labeling of Adherent Target Cells (UV-2237 Fibrosarcoma)

1. UV-2237 target cells are routinely cultured in supplemented CMEM + 5% ΔFBS. One day prior to labeling with [^{3}H]proline, split UV-2237 cells into T-75 tissue culture flasks so as to obtain a 40%-50% confluent monolayer culture 24 hr later.

2. Wash the monolayer culture with CMEM (without nonessential amino acids). Add 0.15 ml of [^{3}H]proline stock and 10 ml of CMEM + 5% ΔFBS (without nonessential amino acids) to the monolayer culture. Incubate for 24 hr.

3. Harvest [^{3}H]proline-labeled cells by treating the monolayer culture with 0.25% trypsin-EDTA in CMF-HBSS for 15-20 sec.

4. Wash cells and resuspend in CMEM + 5% ΔFBS.

5. Perform a cell count and adjust cells to 5 x 10^4/ml in CMEM + 5% ΔFBS.

6. Determine input counts of labeled target cells by solubilizing 10^4 labeled cells in 0.2 ml of 2% Triton-X. Transfer the Triton-X solubilized cell mixture to a scintillation vial, and add 1 ml of scintillation fluid. Determine radioactivity in a beta counter.

Note: Input for labeled cells should be at least 5,000 cpm/10^4 cells.

7. Add 0.2 ml of the 5 x 10^4/ml cell suspension to each well of the 96-well microtiter plate (10^4 cells/well).

8. Incubate plates overnight at 37°C in a humidified incubator with 5% CO$_2$ atmosphere.

9. Add spleen NK cells the next day.

13.404 Preparation of Spleen NK Cells

1. Prepare spleen cells as described under section 6.100.

2. Perform a cell count and adjust the cell concentration to 5 x 10^6 viable cells/ml in CMEM + 5% ΔFBS. Store cells on ice until plated.

13.405 Plating of Long-Term [^{3}H]Proline Assay

1. Aspirate the culture media from the wells of the microtiter plates containing the [^{3}H]proline-labeled target cells.

2. Add 0.2 ml of the appropriate spleen cell suspension (5 x 10^6/ml, 2.5 x 10^6/ml, 1.25 x 10^6/ml, and 0.6 x 10^6/ml) to each well that contains proline-labeled target cells.

Routine plate effector/ target ratios are 100:1, 50:1, 25:1,
and 12:1.

Note: Plate specific spleen cell suspension in triplicate. Be
sure to incubate [^{3}H]proline-labeled targets in medium
alone (medium control wells).

3. Incubate plates for 24 hr at 37°C in a humidified incubator
with 5% CO_2 atmosphere.

4. After the incubation period, wash the wells twice with HBSS.
Aspirate the wells to an almost dry state.

5. Add 0.2 ml of 2% Triton-X to each well. Incubate for 15-20
min at 37°C.

6. Using a different micropipette tip for each triplicate culture
wells, aspirate the Triton-X solubilized cell mixture up and
down three to five times, and transfer the contents to each
well into a scintillation vial.

7. Add 1 ml scintillation fluid to each vial. Cap vials and
monitor radioactivity in a beta scintillation counter.

13.406 Calculation of percent Cytotoxicity

$$1- \left(\frac{\text{cpm remaining in exp. well}}{\text{cpm remaining in medium control well}} \right) \times 100$$

13.500 Determination of the Kinetics of NK Cell Activation and the Potential to Sustain NK Cell Activity

13.501 Kinetics

1. The kinetics of NK cell activity are determined by the sequential injection of the BRM and a single assessment of NK cell
activity.

2. The optimal time points for BRM stimulation are generally days
-14, -10, -7, -4, -3, -2, -1, and, if appropriate, -2 hr
before the harvest of spleens for the assay.

13.502 Sustaining Activity

1. The ability of a BRM to sustain NK cell activity or induce
a NK cell hyporesponsive state is also assessed with spleen
cells from the various groups of mice at a common time point.

2. The appropriate groups include
a) HBSS (negative control)

b) Poly IC day -1 (positive control)

c) BRM administered at peak time point (based on 13.501)

d) BRM administered 1X per week for 2 weeks

e) BRM administered 2X per week for 2 weeks

f) BRM administered daily for 2 weeks

g) MVE-2 administered at day -3 (positive control)

h) MVE-2 administered daily for 2 weeks (positive control)

14.000   MACROPHAGE MICROCYTOTOXICITY ASSAY (46)

14.100   Reagents

CMEM medium + 5% ΔFBS

CMF-HBSS

Trypan blue

Trypsin (0.25%) - EDTA solution in CMF-HBSS

Sodium hydroxide (0.1 M NaOH solution in water)

$[^{125}I]$IUdR (10 μCi/ml)

14.200   Materials

75-cm^2 tissue culture flasks (Costar)

96-well flat-bottom microtiter plates (Costar)

50- and 250-ml conical-bottom centrifuge tubes

12 x 75-mm glass tubes

1-, 5-, 10-ml pipettes; Pasteur pipettes

Microdoser with sterile tips

Hemacytometer

Compound research microscope

Humidified, 5% CO$_2$ incubator

Double-tipped cotton swabs

Refrigerated centrifuges (Beckman TJ-6 and Sorvall)

Gamma counter

14.300   Plating of 72-hr Macrophage Microcytotoxicity Assay

1.   Collect mouse peritoneal macrophages, mouse alveolar macrophages, or rat alveolar macrophages as described in sections
6.300 and 6.400. For in vitro activation, collect macrophages
from normal animals; in vivo activation, collect macrophages
from animals 24 hr after i.v. injection of BRM and controls.

Note: Keep macrophages on ice until plated.

2. Centrifuge macrophages at 1,200 rpm for 6 min and resuspend in serum-free CMEM.

3. Perform a cell count in WBCF and adjust cell suspensions to 7.5 x 10^5 viable cells/ml in CMEM.

4. Plate 0.2 ml (1.5 x 10^5 cells) of each macrophage suspension in triplicate for each in vivo activation. Group triplicate groupings of the macrophage for each BRM dose or control to be used in the in vitro activation. Plating is done in a 96-well flat-bottom microtiter plate.

5. Incubate plates for 1 hr at 37°C in a humidified incubator with 5% CO_2 atmosphere.

6. If the experiment is measuring in vitro activation, aspirate the medium from each well and add the appropriate BRM and controls. Add each agent to three additional wells for a toxicity control. If the experiment measures in vivo activation, the 24-hr agent incubation can be accomplished in vivo and the target cells can be added immediately after the macrophages adhere to the wells.

7. Aspirate the medium from each well and add 2 x 10^4 (rat) or 1 x 10^4 (mouse) labeled target cells in 0.2 ml of CMEM + 5% ΔFBS/well. (Do not aspirate medium from more wells than can be refilled in approximately 1 min.)

Note: For duration of in vitro activation studies, macrophages are incubated with optimal activating dose of a BRM for 24 hr. Following a wash with CMEM + 5% ΔFBS, labeled target cells are added 24, 48, or 96 hr after the 24-hr incubation with BRM.

Note: For studies of the kinetics of in vivo activation, mice are injected on days -4, -3, -2, and -1, and the alveolar macrophages are lavaged on day 0. These macrophages are then used in the routine 72-hr macrophage cytotoxicity assay.

8. Incubate macrophages with labeled target cells for 24 hr at 37°C in a humidified incubator with 5% CO_2 atmosphere.

9. Aspirate off medium from each well and add 0.2 ml fresh CMEM + 5% ΔFBS/well. Incubate for an additional 48 hr.

Note: Negative controls for assay include target cells alone as well as normal macrophage cocultivated with target cells. Positive controls are macrophages incubated with 5 µg/ml LPS, MLV incorporating MTP-PE, or poly ICLC.

14.400 Harvesting of 72-hr Microcytotoxicity Assay

1. Be sure plates are marked so that the identification of each test triplicate is known when lids are removed.

2. Aspirate the medium from the wells of all plates.

3. Add 0.2 ml of CMF-HBSS to each well.

4. Aspirate the CMF-HBSS from the wells of all plates.

5. Using a microdoser pipette, add 0.1 ml of 0.1 M NaOH to each well. Incubate plates at 37°C for 20 min. Following incubation, randomly check the contents of control target wells microscopically to be sure cells are lysed. If cells are not completely lysed, incubate at 37°C until complete lysis occurs.

6. Place individual cotton swabs (Q Tips) in each well. Allow the cotton to absorb the NaOH-cell lysate mixture and then swab the bottom of each well vigorously. Transfer each radioactive swab to a 12 x 75-mm glass tube and place in a gamma counter.

14.500 Calculation of Percent Cytotoxicity (Using mean value of triplicates)

$$\left(\frac{\text{cpm in control group - cpm experimental group}}{\text{cpm control group}}\right) \times 100$$

14.600 ^{111}In Labeling of Target Cells (47)

See section 4.604 using P815 or L5178Y as target cells.

14.700 Plating of ^{111}In Release Macrophage Microcytotoxicity Assay

1. Collect mouse peritoneal macrophages, alveolar macrophages, Kupffer cells, or rat alveolar macrophages as described in sections 6.200 and 6.500. For in vitro activation, collect

macrophages from normal animals; for in vivo activation, collect macrophages from animals 24 hr after i.v. injection of BRM or control substances.

Note: Keep macrophages on ice until plated.

2. Centrifuge macrophages at 1,200 rpm for a 6 min and resuspend in serum-free medium.

3. Perform a cell count in WBCF and adjust cell suspensions to 10.0×10^5 viable cells/ml in CMEM.

4. Plate 0.2 ml (2×10^5 cells) of each macrophage suspension in triplicate for each in vivo activation group or triplicate groupings of the macrophage for each BRM dose or control to be used in the in vitro activation. Plating is done in a 96-well flat-bottom microtiter plate.

5. Incubate plates for 1 hr at 37°C in a humidified incubator with 5% CO_2 atmosphere.

6. If the experiment measures in vitro activation, aspirate the medium from each well and add the appropriate BRM. Add each dilution to three additional wells. If the experiment measures in vivo activation, the 24-hr agent incubation was accomplished in vivo and the target cells can be added immediately after adherence of macrophages.

7. Aspirate the medium from each well and add 2×10^4 (rat) or 1×10^4 (mouse) labeled target cells in 0.2 ml of CMEM + 5% ΔFBS/well. (Do not aspirate medium from more wells than can be refilled in approximately 1 min.)

Note: For duration of in vitro activation studies, macrophages are incubated with optimal activating dose of a BRM for 24 hr. Following a wash with CMEM + 5% ΔFBS, labeled target cells are added 24, 48, or 96 hr after incubation with BRM.

Note: For studies of the kinetics of in vivo activation, mice are injected on days -10, -7, -4, -3, -2, and -1 and the alveola macrophages are lavaged on day 0. These macrophages are the used in the routine 72-hr macrophage cytotoxicity assay.

8. Incubate macrophages with labeled target cells for 18 hr at 37° in a humidified incubator with 5% CO_2 atmosphere for suspension cell targets (P815 or L51784) or 48 hr for adherent targets.

Note: Negative controls for the assay include target cells incubated alone as well as normal macrophages cocultivated with target cells. Positive controls are macrophages incubated with 5 µg/ml LPS, MLV incorporating MTP-PE, or poly ICLC.

14.800 Harvesting of ^{111}In Release Microcytotoxicity Assay

1. Be sure plates are marked so that the identification of each test triplicate is known when lids are removed.
2. Centrifuge the plate for 3 min at 600 rpm.
3. Gently remove 100 microliters of supernate/well.
4. To obtain total release, incubate cells with 100 microliters of triton-X 100.

14.900 Calculation of Percent Cytotoxicity (Using mean value of triplicates)

$$\frac{\text{cpm in experimental group - cpm control group}}{\text{cpm total release group}} \times 100$$

15.000 B-CELL ASSAYS

15.100 Hemagglutination Assay

The hemagglutination assay measures both the primary antibody response (IgM) and the secondary antibody response (IgG).

15.101 Reagents

HBSS

Fresh SRBC in Alsever's solution

15.102 Materials

15-, 50-ml conical tubes

25-gauge needle, 1-cc syringe

1-, 5-, and 10-ml pipettes

Pasteur pipette

12 x 75-mm glass tube

15.103 Procedures

1. Place 2-5 ml of SRBC in Alsever's solution in a 50-ml conical tube. Wash the SRBC 3X in HBSS. This is done by adding PBS to the tube of SRBC to bring the volume to 50 ml. Centrifuge the tube at ~400 x g for 5 min, discard the supernatant, and resuspend the SRBC in 50 ml of PBS. After the final

wash, resuspend the SRBC in PBS at a 2.5% v/v suspension ($\sim$5 x 10^8 cells/ml).

2. Immunize 8- to 12-wk-old C57BL/6 mice with $\sim 10^8$ SRBC (0.2 ml) by i.p. injection.

3. Inject the BRM at various dilutions i.v. either concomitantly or 1 to 4 days after the injection of the SRBC.

4. Bleed mice, including control animals injected with HBSS or SRBC, from the retinal orbital plexus 5 days, 7 days, 10 days, 14 days, and 20 days following challenge with SRBC.

5. Bleed the mice individually and store their sera at -70°C in Eppendorf tubes until used in the hemagglutination assay.

15.200 Murine Lymphocyte Proliferation Assay

15.201 Reagents

RPMI-1640

HEPES-1-M

Gentamicin, 50 µg/ml

L-Glutamine, 200 mM

ΔFBS (50°C, -30')

PWM

LPS

15.202 Materials

15-, 50-ml conical tubes

1-, 5-, 10-ml pipettes

96-well flat-bottom microtiter plate

15.203 Procedure

1. Inject 8- to 12-wk-old BALB/c mice i.v. with BRM.

2. Prepare single-cell suspensions of spleens and resuspend in 10 ml of RPMI-1640 (500 ml) supplemented with HEPES (25 mM), gentamicin (50 µg), L-glutamine (1%), and FBS (10%).

3. Determine the viable cell numbers.

4. Centrifuge the tube at $\sim$200 x g for 10 min. Discard the supernatant fluid and resuspend the cell pellet to a concentration of 2-2.5 x 10^6 cells/ml with the media described above.

5. Add 0.1 ml of the cell suspension to replicate wells of a flat-bottom microtiter plate.

6. Add concentrations of T-cell-dependent B-cell mitogen (PWM) or T-cell-independent B-cell mitogen (LPS) in 0.1-ml vol to appropriate replicate wells.

7. Incubate cultures for 3 days at 37°C in a humidified incubator with 5% CO_2 atmosphere.

8. Add 2.0 μCi [^{3}H]thymidine in 0.025-ml vol to each well 16 hr prior to the termination of the cultures.

9. Harvest the cells with a multiple sample harvester onto strips of fiberglass paper and determine the labeled DNA by liquid scintillation spectroscopy by counting for at least 1 min.

10. Mitogen response data from lymphocytes of treated animals are expressed as cpm. Data are also expressed as a RPI, which is the ratio of response in treated animals net cpm relative to mean in control animals. The data are also expressed as percentage of change (% change) in the treatment groups relative to nontreated controls:

net cpm = cpm in mitogen culture - in control cultures

$$\% \text{ change} = 1 - \frac{\text{net cpm in treated} \times 100}{\text{net cpm in untreated animal}}$$

15.300 Vivo-Vivo Adjuvant activity for B cells (Enzyme-Linked Immunosorbent (Assay)

15.301 Reagents

Bovine serum albumin (1 mg/ml HBSS)

PBS - Tween 80

Coating buffer (carbonate buffer with BSA 25 μg/ml)

Washing buffer (PBS-Tween 80)

Substrate buffer (10% diethanolamine buffer)

Phosphatase substrate tablets (p-nitro-phenyldisodium phosphate)

Stop buffer (3 M NaOH)

Developing antibody, alkaline phosphatase-conjugated antimouse IgG

15.302 Materials

U-bottom, 96-well ELISA plates

P-200 ml micropipette aid

Microdoser and tips

25-gauge hypodermic needles

1-cc syringes

1-, 2-, 5-, and 10-ml pipettes

15.303   Immunization and Serum Collection

1. Immunize C57BL-6 mice (i.p.) on day 0 with 500 µg BSA in HBSS (0.5 ml) per mouse.

2. Inject the BRM i.p. on day 0 or day +2.

3. Collect blood (0.2-.03 ml) from the retro-orbital plexus (see 3.904) of each mouse with a glass pipette and place individually in a 1-cc centrifuge tube.

4. Centrifuge blood at 1,800 rpm for 8 min.

5. Aspirate serum and store in marked centrifuge tubes at -70°C.

6. Bleed the mice sequentially, including a prebleed and on days 4, 7, 10, 14, 21, 28, and 35.

15.304   ELISA Assay

1. Coat 96-well U-bottom ELISA plates with BSA (5 µg/well) in coating buffer and incubate at 37°C (overnight). Store at 4°C until the day of the test. Use within 4 days.

2. Wash plates three times use with PBS-Tween 80.

3. Pool aliquots (10 µl) of sera from five individual mice per group.

4. Dilute sera pools from 1:20, using serial $\log_2$ dilutions to 1:80,000 with PBS-Tween 80. Do not use any dilution less than 1:20 to avoid a prozone effect.

5. Dispense samples in 0.1-ml aliquots to appropriate wells.

6. Incubate plates for 1 hr at 37°C.

7. Wash plates three times with PBS-Tween 80.

8. Add conjugated IgG (1:2,000 dilution in PBS-Tween 80) 0.1-ml aliquots per well.

9. Incubate plates at 37°C for 1 hr.

10. Wash plates three times with PBS-Tween 80.

11. Dispense substrate (one phosphatase substrate tablet in 5 ml 10% diethanolamine buffer) in 0.1-ml aliquots into wells.

12. Incubate plates at 37°C for 30 minutes.

13. Add stop solution (0.05-ml of 3 M NaOH) to wells, including one uncoated/untreated well for blank.
14. Read plates in ELISA reader.

16.000 BRIEF REVIEW OF IMMUNOMODULATORY PROTOCOLS

16.100 T-Lymphocyte Assays

The in vitro assays employed to monitor T-lymphocyte activity include the following:

1. A one-way, syngeneic MLR utilizing C57BL/6 mouse splenic lymphocytes as responders and C3H⁻ spleen cells (X-irridiated) as stimulators. Cell proliferation is monitored by assaying DNA synthesis via incorporation of [^{3}H]thymidine.

2. An allogeneic MLTR-CMC utilizing C3H⁻ mouse splenic lymphocytes as responders and P815 tumor cells (X-irradiated) as stimulators. The in vitro generation of cytotoxic T lymphocytes is monitored by the ability of the incubated lymphocytes to lyse P815 tumor cells in a tumor-specific manner.

3. A quantitative assay of tumor-specific cytolytic T-lymphocyte activity (CTL) is measured by radioactive release from pre-labeled syngeneic target cells.

4. A mitogen-induced blastogenesis assay in which mouse splenic lymphocytes are cultured in optimal doses of concanavalin A and various dilutions of BRM. Cell proliferation is monitored by assaying DNA synthesis via incorporation of [^{3}H]thymidine. This provides information regarding the mechanism of inhibition in the MLTR, e.g., toxicity or inhibition of proliferation.

5. Direct determination of lymphocyte viability in MLR or MLTR assays using viability staining and fluorescence microscopy

6. Where a decrease in MLTR-CMC or CTL response does not inhibit the concanavalin A stimulation of lymphocytes this suggest that the immunomodulator should be tested for the induction of suppressor cell activity. This is accomplished by removing the lymphocytes from the MLTR cultures on day 5 and adding graded doses of these cells, after extensive washing, to a MLR or MLTR-CMC assay.

7. Those BRM which stimulated MLTR-CMC or CTL responses can be tested for helper cell activity. This is accomplished by removing the lymphocytes from the MLTR cultures and adding graded doses of these lymphocytes to a MLR or MLTR-CMC assay. The ability of the cells to stimulate the normal lymphocyte response in a tumor-antigen specific manner will be determined.

8. The nature of the effector cell and the regulator cell are determined using antiserum-complement depletion studies with anti-Thy-1, anti-asialo GM1; and anti-Lyt 1, 2, or 3 antiserum.

16.101 In Vitro Activation: In Vitro Testing
Test Animals: 6- to 8-wk-old C3H-mice

1. The ability of a BRM to affect T lymphocyte responsiveness in vitro is assessed by first incorporating five different doses of a BRM into a one-way MLR assay system. Mouse splenic lymphocytes (responders) are cultured with X-irradiated C3H-spleen cell (stimulators) at a responder/stimulator ratio of 10:1 either alone or with BRM for 3 or 4 days. Representative samples of the cultures are pulsed with [^{3}H]thymidine for 24 hr to monitor DNA synthesis.

2. Further evidence for the ability of a BRM to modulate T lymphocyte activity can be obtained by the addition of five different doses of a BRM to the MLTR culture system. Mouse splenic lymphocytes (responders) are cultured with X-irradiated P815 tumor cells (stimulators) at a responder/stimulator ratio of 300:1 either alone or with BRM for 5 days. On day 5, representative samples of cultured lymphocytes are tested for their ability to lyse the tumor cells using a radiolabel release assay. Effector cell/target ratios are 50:1, 25:1, 12:1, 6:1.

3. BRM-induced suppression/stimulation which was revealed by either the MLR or MLTR test systems can be further analyzed by incubating normal splenic lymphocytes with a BRM and then adding the BRMstimulated cells to the MLR and MLTR systems. BRM-induced regulator cells added to these cultures should

affect cell proliferation (MLR) or the generation of cytotoxic lymphocytes (MLTR), respectively.

16.102   In Vivo Activation: In Vitro Testing

Test Animals: 8-wk-old C3H⁻ mice.

1. The ability of a BRM to augment the in vivo generation of tumor-specific cytotoxic cells is evaluated in the following manner. Mice are immunized at five i.d. sites in the belly region with 5×10^6 viable UV-2237 tumor cells either alone or admixed with three different doses of a BRM. Tumor cells used to immunize are obtained by the collagenase dissociation of nonnecrotic tumors growing s.c. These cells are stored in liquid nitrogen and X-irradiated just before use. Untreated mice and mice treated with BRM alone serve as controls. Ten days after immunization, half the mice in each group are killed and their spleens or regional lymph nodes assessed for the presence of cytotoxic lymphocytes in a radiolabeled release assay using specific and non-crossreactive labeled cells. Effector cell/target cell ratios are 200:1, 100:1, 50:1, and 25:1.

2. A secondary cytotoxic lymphocyte response is assessed by injecting the remaining immunized mice on day 10 with 2×10^6 viable UV-2237 fibrosarcoma or K-1735 melanoma (non-cross-reactive) cells at two i.d. sites in the abdominal region. Tumor cells used to immunize are obtained by collagenase dissociation of nonnecrotic s.c. tumors. These cells are stored in liquid nitrogen and X-irradiated just before use. Five days following the second immunization (15 days after initial immunization), the mice are killed and their spleens or regional lymph nodes cells harvested and tested against specific and non-crossreactive radiolabeled target cells at effector cell/target cell ratios of 200:1, 100:1, 50:1, and 25:1.

16.200   B-Cell Assays

The in vitro assays employed to monitor B-lymphocyte activity are the following:

1. Serum hemagglutination assay

2. A blastogenic response to PWM and LPS stimulation

3. ELISA assay of serum antibody levels to BSA

16.201 In Vitro Activation:In Vitro Testing

None are specified.

16.202 In Vivo Activation:In Vitro Testing

Test Animals: 8- to 12-wk-old BALB/c mice

1. The ability of a BRM to augment the in vivo generation of primary antibody (IgM) and secondary antibody. The immunogen is injected i.p. and the BRM administered 24-96 hr later. Mice are tail bled at several time points thereafter and the antibody levels determined by hemagglutination or ELISA assay.

2. The BRM are injected i.v. and the spleen cells are removed at various time points. The ability of the cells to respond to the T-cell-dependent B-cell mitogen, PWM, and the T-cell-independent B-cell mitogen, LPS, is determined in a micro-blastogenesis assay. The cultures are harvested at 72 hr following a 6- to 8-hr [^{3}H]thymidine pulse.

16.300 Natural Killer (NK) Cell Assays

The in vitro cytotoxicity assay for measuring NK cell killing is the 4-hr ^{51}Cr-release assay from labeled YAC lymphoma target cells.

16.301 In Vitro Activation:In Vitro Testing

Test Animals: 3-wk-old weanling C3H⁻ mice.

1. In vitro activation of NK cells is studied by incubating normal spleen cells with BRM at five different doses for 24 hr. The requirements for the in vitro activation of NK cells by the different agents, e.g., direct activation by reacting with NK or pre-NK cells or indirect activation by macrophage stimulation and production of interferon may be assessed by incubation with anti-interferon. NK activity is assessed by the 4-hr ^{51}Cr labeled assay with YAC cells as targets.

16.302 In Vivo Activation:In Vitro Testing

Test Animals: 3-wk-old C3H⁻ mice

1. BRM at five different doses are injected i.v. into recipient mice. The in vitro activity of NK cells 1 to 10 days after treatment is determined by the 4-hr ^{51}Cr-YAC release assay.

2. Levels of interferon in the blood of recipient mice are measured 24 hr after i.v. treatment.

16.400 Macrophage Assays

The in vitro cytotoxicity assay is a 72-hr microcytotoxicity assay and is based on the radiorelease (cytolysis) of $[^{125}I]IUdR$-labeled B16 tumor target cells. Alternatively a 24-hr (suspension cell targets) or 48-hr (adherent targets) ^{111}In release assay may also be used. Suspension cell targets are P815 or L5178Y lymphoma cells.

1. For mouse alveolar macrophages, the B16-BL6 melanoma serve as target.

2. For rat alveolar macrophages, the F344 mammary adenocarcinoma 200 serves as target.

16.401 In Vitro Activation:In Vitro Testing

Test Animals: 6- to 8-wk-old C57BL/6 mice and 12- to 16-wk-old F344 rats

1. In order to determine the optimal dose of a BRM for maximal in vitro macrophage activation, mouse AM and/or rat AM from normal animals are incubated for 24 hr with a BRM (at five different doses). The macrophages are then washed and labeled target cells are added (72-hr microcytotoxicity assay).

2. Once the optimal dose of BRM necessary to obtain maximal activation in vitro is known, it is tested for its ability to maintain macrophage-tumoricidal properties (duration of activated state). Normal mouse AM and/or rat AM are incubated with the optimal dose of a BRM for 24 hr and then washed. Labeled target cells are added 24, 48, 96, or 168 hr after incubation with BRM. The tumoricidal capacity of the macrophages is then assessed by a 72-hr microcytotoxicity assay.

16.402 In Vivo Activation:In Vitro Testing

Test Animals: 6- to 8-wk-old C57BL/6 mice and 8- to 12-wk-old F344 rats.

1. In order to determine the optimal dose of a BRM for maximal in vivo macrophage activation, a BRM is injected at several different doses i.v. into mice and rats. Routinely mouse PM and AM rat are harvested 24 hr after systemic adminis-

tration of the BRM. Macrophage tumoricidal activity is determined in vitro in an assay against [^{125}I] IUdR-labeled target cells in a 72-hr microcytotoxicity assay.

17.000 THERAPY MODELS OF TRANSPLANTABLE TUMORS (48,49)

The preclinical evaluation of BRM agents for the treatment of cancer requires the testing of these agents with the use of relevant in vivo model systems. The experimental tumor models listed below are directly applicable to this goal. Both transplantable tumor systems and primary autochthonous hosts are used to evaluate the therapeutic efficacy of BRMs.

Transplantable Neoplasms

Tumor	Host(mice)	Initiating Dose	Size at Resectio
B16-BL6	C57BL/6	5×10^4	8-10 mm
UV-2237	C3H-	1×10^5	-
UV-2237 mm (parent)	C3H-	1×10^5 or 5×10^4	12-15 mm
UV-2237 cl 46 or UV-2240	UV-irradiated C3H-	2×10^5	-
MCA 3152	C3H	1×10^5	-
K1735 mm	C3H	1×10^5	12-15 mm
M109	BALB/c	1×10^5	8-10 mm
3LL	C57BL/6	1×10^5	12-15 mm

All the neoplasms listed above are spontaneously metastatic as well as capable of forming lung colonies. Tumors are injected at a "primary site" and surgically removed when they have reached an appropriate size. Multiple treatments with BRM begins 48-72 hr after resection of the primary neoplasm. The time to death in each tumor system is sufficiently long to allow for multiple treatments. All BRM agents are administered i.v. The schedule of BRM treatment and dose will be based on the data obtained in the in vivo activation: in vitro testing portion of the screen.

Two types of therapy studies are performed: (1) Tumor-bearing animals are killed 10-12 wk after initiation of the primary tumor. The presence or absence of metastatic tumor foci following BRM treatment are assessed by gross and microscopic examination of target organs. (2) Those BRMs found to be of therapeutic benefit in the short 10- to 12-wk assay are tested in lifetime survival studies.

17.100 Adjuvant Activity of the BRM: Induction of a Specific Cytotoxic T-Cell Response

Test Animals: 6- to 8-wk-old C3H⁻ mice

1. The ability of a BRM to affect immunization-induced resistance to a tumor challenge implant is studied with two antigenically unrelated tumors designated K-1735 mm melanoma and UV-2237 fibrosarcoma (progressively growing tumors in normal mice). Mice are immunized i.d. in the abdominal region with 1×10^6 X-irradiated (10,000 rad) UV-2237 cells, either alone, with three different doses of a BRM, or with the BRM alone. Tumor cells used to immunize are obtained by the collagenase dissociation of nonnecrotic s.c. tumors. These cells are stored in liquid nitrogen and X-irradiated before use. Tumor challenge is accomplished by footpad injection with 1×10^5 viable parent K-1735 mm cells or 1×10^5 viable UV-2237 cells. Tumor incidence and growth rates are monitored once weekly for 4-6 wk.

17.200 Ability of a BRM to Stimulate Effector T-Cell Activation in the Presence of Suppressor T Cells

In order to determine if a specific BRM treatment is capable of altering the growth of a UV-radiation-induced tumor in a UV-irradiated host, the following studies are performed. Mice exposed to chronic UV radiation (3X/wk for 12 wk) are immunized with three different doses of a BRM, three different doses of a BRM admixed with 5×10^6 collagenase-dissociated tumor cells, or 5×10^6 collagenase-dissociated tumor cells alone. Immunization is accomplished by five i.d. administration sites. These groups are challenged, as well as control UV-irradiated mice and normal mice, with 10^5 tumor cells (UV-2237 clone 46) injected into the footpad.

17.300 Ability of a BRM to Activate Nonspecific Effector NK Cells In Vivo and Inhibit the Formation of Pulmonary Tumor Nodules

Test Animals: 3-wk-old C3H⁻ mice

1. Five different doses of a BRM are injected i.v. 48 hr before the i.v. injection of 5×10^4 UV-2237 mm cells into 3-wk-old weanling C3H⁻ mice. The prevention of experimental metastasis (presumably by activation of NK cells) can be determined in this study.

17.400 Therapy of Established Secondary Tumors

The preclinical evaluation of BRM agents for the treatment of cancer requires the development of relevant in vivo models. Obviously, the optimal therapeutic model should closely approximate the clinical reality, e.g., the initiation of therapy against established secondary disease after surgical intervention. The efficacy of such a model is then determined, based on long-term survival. Thus, an optimal animal model would involve approximately a 9- to 12-mo assay. A simplification of this assay entails the necropsy of mice following the therapeutic regimen and determination of metastatic burden.

In general, the assays use tumors injected at a "primary site" and surgically removed when they have reached an appropriate size (resulting in >90% incidence of spontaneous metastases). Repeated i.v. treatments with BRM start 72 hr after resection of the primary neoplasm. The time to death in each tumor system should be of sufficient time to allow for multiple treatments (4-6 weeks).

Thus, therapy studies can be terminated to achieve two types of evaluations: (1) tumor-bearing animals are killed 10-12 wk following initiation of the primary tumor and the presence or absence of metastatic tumor foci following BRM treatment assessed by gross and microscopic examination of target organs and (2) the BRM agents are tested in a lifetime survival studies.

Another and more rapid determination of therapeutic efficacy is based on experimental metastases. This assay comprises a model in which i.v. injected tumor cells are used to establish tumor foci and differs from models in which the primary tumors were resected tumors in that i.v. injected mice are not "conditioned" by the primary tumor burden. Furthermore, the experimental metastasis assay provides a highly reproducible, tumor burden. A positive response is based on a reduction in the percent of tumor free mice, the median number of pulmonary tumor foci, and/or in the median survival time.

17.401 Testing Protocol

Test Animals: 6- to 8 wk-old C57BL/6 mice

1. BRM agents are injected i.v. into mice bearing the spontaneously metastatic B16-BL6 melanoma (tumors are induced by injection at a primary site and then surgically removed). The ability of a
BRM to eradicate established metastases is determined by beginning treatment with a BRM 72 hr following the surgical removal of primary tumors.

2. Therapeutic efficiency is determined from the percentage of mice "cured" of their tumor, median (range) of pulmonary tumor foci, and median survival time.

3. Data are obtained by performing necropsies on morbid mice, fixing metastasis-bearing organs, and noting the date of death. Mice surviving 45 days after the last control mouse has died are killed and necropsied. The presence of tumor burden must then be determined.

4. All initial therapy protocols use a treatment regimen of twice weekly injections of the BRM for 4 weeks.

18.000 TESTING OF BRMS IN AUTOCHTHONOUS TUMOR MODELS (48,49)

BRMs are tested in UV-irradiated mice bearing autochthonous neoplasms and in rats with N-methyl-N-nitrosourea (NMU) induced mammary tumors.

18.100 UV Carcinogenesis

Test Animals: 6-wk-old BALB/c mice

The skin tumors induced in mice by chronic UV-irradiation (fibrosarcoma, rhabdomyosarcomas, hemangosarcomas, and squamous cell carcinomas) are often highly antigenic and exhibit individual as well as common antigenic specificities when tested by in vivo

transplantation techniques or <u>in vitro</u> cytotoxicity assays.
These skin tumors differ from those induced by chemical carcinogens in that the majority are rejected following transplantation
to normal syngeneic mice but grow progressively in immunosuppressed recipients or in mice exposed to chronic, subtumorigenic
(2 months) UV irradiation. Prior to the development of primary
UV-induced tumors, unirradiated mice lose their ability to reject
transplants of regressor UV-induced tumors by a mechanism that
involves T-cell-mediated immunosuppression. This immunological
hyporesponsiveness extends to all syngeneic UV-induced tumors
but not to other non-UV-induced tumors. The immunological aspect of this systemic alteration can be adoptively transferred
with lymphoid cells from UV-irradiated mice to lethally irradiated
normal recipients. The suppressor T cells express membrane associated Thy 1, and Ia antigens and are X-radiation sensitive.

A second immunologic perturbation in UV-irradiated mice is
an alteration in the presentation of certain antigens. This
immunologic deficiency is expressed as an inability of the mice
to serve as recipients in a local graft-versus-host reaction
and to develop a delayed hypersensitivity response against contact allergens. Recent results have demonstrated that antigen-
presenting cells (macrophages or Langerhans cells from the
spleen or skin, respectively) of UV-irradiated mice are func-
tionally altered. However, the inability of UV-irradiated mice
to mount a contact hypersensitivity reaction can be overcome by
introducing the antigens on normal antigen presenting cells, suggesting that the UV-irradiated mice have a normal lymphocyte
response. Furthermore, induction by the UV exposure of altered
antigen presenting cells (for contact hypersensitivity) also
results in the induction of antigenspecific suppressor T cells.
The current hypothesis suggests that the UV-mediated alterations
in antigen-presenting cells results in specific immunosuppression
probably by the induction of a suppressor cell.

The radiation source is a bank of six Westinghouse FS40 sun-
lamps that should deliver an average dose rate of 2.8 $J/m^2/sec$
over the wavelength range of 280-340 nm. This output cannot be

assumed but must be periodically measured. Five mice are housed per cage on a shelf 20 cm below the lamps, and the cage order is systematically rotated before each treatment to compensate for the uneven lamp output along the shelf. The mice are irradiated for 2 hr three times per week (Monday, Wednesday, Friday) for a minimum of 3 mo before their use. To induce autochthonous tumors, irradiation is continued until the appearance of the first tumors. In this strain the time to first appearance for this regimen of UV irradiation is approximately 32 wk, with a range of 22-42 wk (tumors appear earlier in BALB/c mice). Multiple UV-radiation-induced tumors appear mainly on the ears. Systemic immunotherapy (i.v. injection) is individually initiated at the first appearance of a primary tumor (approximately 1-2 mm in diameter). Intra-lesional therapy is initiated when the lesions are approximately 4-6 mm in diameter and consists of a single treatment in a volume of 0.05 ml. The schedule and dose of BRM treatment are derived from data of the in vivo activation: in vitro testing portion of the screen and is continued for 4 weeks. Therapeutic efficacy is determined by the ability of a BRM to retard the development of the primary tumor or eradicate the primary tumor after dilution and prevent the development of other primary tumors. Because these control treated UV-induced primary tumors have a 20-30% incidence of metastasis, the incidence of grossly observable and histiologically evident secondary disease is also determined. The tumor volumes are determined weekly by measuring the tumor diameter in two dimensions. The formula $V = 0.5 \times a \times b^2$, where a = the large diameter and b = the smaller diameter, is used to calculate the volume. Each individual growth curve is fitted to a Gompertz curve and then the curves from each group are combined statistically. Survival data are analyzed using the non-parametric Kruskal-Wallis analysis as adapted for censored observations by Gehan and Breslow and the Cox proportional hazards model. Both these analyses require at least 20 animals per group.

18.200 NMU Carcinogenesis

Test Animals: 50-day-old virgin female Sprague Dawley rats

A single i.v. or s.c. injection of NMU rapidly and repro-

ducibly induces mammary tumors in a high percentage of rats.
The kinetics of tumor development and the extent (both number
of animals with tumors and the number of tumors per animal) of
tumors is dosage dependent. Animals that receive lower doses
of NMU (~30 mg/kg) develop approximately a 30% incidence of pulmonary metastasis. The rate of development of both primary
tumors as well as the extent of metastasis is strain dependent.

A single i.v. dose of NMU (30-50 mg/kg) is administered to
50-day-old female Sprague Dawley rats. NMU stability is dependent
on both temperature and pH. Therefore, dose should be confirmed
by UV spectrometry both before and after injection. This treatment results in the induction of spontaneous mammary adenocarci-
nomas in a high percentage of the animals within 3-4 mo. BRM
treatment is initiated when the primary tumor has grown to a
size of 10-15 mm. For each BRM, three different doses in three
different regimens of treatment are evaluated. All tumor-bearing
rats are weighed and monitored weekly for evidence of a therapeutic effect against tumors. Successfully treated rats are held
for long-term survival and monitored (approximately 1 year) for
the development of metastases.

19.000 POSITIVE CONTROLS

19.100 <u>T-Cell Assays</u>

    MLR: thymosin F5 (100 µg/ml)

    MLTR: thymosin F5 (100 µg/ml)

    CTL: poly ICLC (5 µg/site) or thymosin F5 (500 µg/mouse)

    Therapy: - Thymosin $\alpha 1$ (500 µg/mouse)

                Poly ICLC (3 µg/site)

19.200 <u>NK Cell</u>

    <u>In vitro:in vitro</u>, poly I:C (5 µg/ml)

    <u>In vivo:in vitro</u>, poly I:C (5 µg/mouse)

    <u>In vivo:in vivo</u>, poly I:C (5 µg/mouse)

19.300 <u>Macrophage</u>

    <u>In vitro:in vitro</u>, MTP-PE in MLV, LPS or poly IC

    <u>In vivo:in vitro</u>, MTP-PE in MLV, poly ICLC

19.400 <u>B Cell</u>

    MVE-2

19.500 Therapy

    Poly ICLC, MTP-PE in MLV

APPENDIX

Representative Surface Areas and Weights for Various Species (49)

Species	Body weight (kg)	Surface Area (M^2)
Mouse	0.02	0.0066
Rat	0.15	0.025
Human (adult)	60.0	1.6

Interspecies dosage equivalence conversion

From mg/kg in:
```
   Mouse (20 g)     x  3.0
   Rat (150 g)      x  5.9
   Monkey (3 kg)    x 12.3    = mg/M²
```

Adult (60 kg) x 37.0

From mg/M^2
```
                               x 0.33 = mg/kg in mouse
                               x 0.17 = mg/kg in rat
                               x 0.08 = mg/kg in monkey
                               x 0.03 = mg/kg in human (adult)
```

From mg/kg in mouse
```
                               x 0.50 = mg/kg in rat
                               x 0.24 = mg/kg in monkey
                               x 0.08 = mg/kg in human (adult)
```

From mg/kg in rat
```
                               x 1.97 = mg/kg in mouse
                               x 0.48 = mg/kg in monkey
                               x 0.16 = mg/kg in human (adult)
```

From mg/kg in monkey
```
                               x 4.10 = mg/kg in mouse
                               x 2.08 = mg/kg in rat
                               x 0.33 = mg/kg in human (adult)
```

From mg/kg in human (adult)
```
                               x12.33 = mg/kg in mouse
                               x 6.27 = mg/kg in rat
                               x 3.01 = mg/kg in monkey
```

Decay Table for ^{111}In Ox (half-life, 2.8 days)

Time (hr)	Decay	Time (hr)	Decay
-48	1.642	96	0.370
-36	1.451	108	0.327
-24	1.282	120	0.289
-12	1.132	132	0.255
0	1.000	144	0.226
12	0.883	156	0.199
24	0.780	168	0.176
36	0.689	180	0.156
48	0.609	192	0.138
60	0.538	204	0.122
72	0.475	216	0.108
84	0.419		

Decay Table for ^{125}I (half-life, 60.0 days)

	0	2	4	6	8	10	12	14	16	18
0	-	977	955	933	912	891	871	851	831	812
20	794	776	758	741	724	707	691	675	660	645
40	630	616	602	588	574	561	548	536	524	512
60	500	489	477	467	456	445	435	425	416	406

Decay Table for Chromium-51 (half-life, 27.8 days)

Days	Hours			
	0	6	12	18
0	1.0000	.9938	.9876	.9815
1	.9754	.9693	.9633	.9573
2	.9514	.9454	.9396	.9337
3	.9279	.9222	.9164	.9107
4	.9051	.8995	.8939	.8883
5	.8828	.8773	.8719	.8664
6	.8611	.8557	.8504	.8451
7	.8398	.8346	.8294	.8243
8	.8192	.8141	.8090	.8040
9	.7990	.7940	.7891	.7842
10	.7793	.7745	.7697	.7649
11	.7601	.7554	.7507	.7460
12	.7414	.7368	.7322	.7277
13	.7232	.7187	.7142	.7098
14	.7053	.7010	.6966	.6923
15	.6880	.6837	.6795	.6752
16	.6710	.6669	.6627	.6586
17	.6545	.6504	.6464	.6424
18	.6384	.6344	.6305	.6266
19	.6227	.6188	.6150	.6111
20	.6073	.6036	.5998	.5961
21	.5924	.5887	.5850	.5814
22	.5778	.5742	.5706	.5671
23	.5636	.5601	.5566	.5531
24	.5497	.5463	.5429	.5395
25	.5362	.5328	.5295	.5262
26	.5230	.5197	.5165	.5133
27	.5101	.5069	.5038	.5006
28	.4975	.4944	.4913	.4883
29	.4853	.4822	.4792	.4763

Decay Table for Selenium -75 (half-life, 120.4 days)

Days	Hours									
	0	1	2	3	4	5	6	7	8	9
0	1.0000	.9943	.9886	.9829	.9772	.9716	.9660	.9605	.9550	.9495
10	.9441	.9386	.9332	.9279	.9226	.9173	.9120	.9068	.9016	.8964
20	.8912	.8861	.8810	.8760	.8710	.8660	.8610	.8560	.8511	.8462
1 mo	.8414	.8366	.8317	.8270	.8222	.8175	.8128	.8081	.8035	.7989
10	.7943	.7898	.7852	.7807	.7762	.7718	.7673	.7629	.7586	.7542
20	.7499	.7456	.7413	.7370	.7328	.7286	.7244	.7203	.7161	.7120
2 mo	.7079	.7039	.6998	.6958	.6918	.6878	.6839	.6800	.6761	.6722
10	.6683	.6645	.6607	.6569	.6531	.6494	.6456	.6419	.6382	.6346
20	.6309	.6273	.6237	.6201	.6166	.6130	.6095	.6060	.6025	.5991
3 mo	.5956	.5922	.5888	.5854	.5821	.5787	.5754	.5721	.5688	.5656

REFERENCES

1. Giard, D.J., Aaronson, S.A., Todaro, G.J., Arnstein, P., Kersey, J.H., Dosik, H. and Parks W.P. J. Natl. Cancer Inst. 51, 1417-1423, 1973.
2. Lozzio, C.B. and Lozzio, B.B. J. Natl. Cancer Inst. 50, 535-538, 1973.
3. Sone, S. and Fidler, I.J. Cell. Immunol. 57, 42-50, 1981.
4. Hart, I.R. Am. J. Pathol. 97, 587, 1979.
5. Dunn, T.B. and Potter, M.J. J. Natl. Cancer Inst. 18, 587, 1957.
6. Klein, E. and Klein, G. J. Natl. Cancer Inst. 32, 547, 1964.
7. Kripke, M.L. Cancer Res. 37, 1395, 1977.
8. Kripke, M.L., Gruys, E. and Fidler, I.J. Cancer Res. 38, 2962-2967, 1978.
9. Talmadge, J.E. and Fidler, I.J. J. Natl. Cancer Inst. 69, 975-980, 1982.
10. Fidler, I.J., Gruys, E., Cifone, M.A., Barnes, Z. and Bucana, C. J. Natl. Cancer Inst. 67, 947-956, 1981.
11. Sugiura, K. and Stock, C.C. Cancer Res. 15, 38-45, 1955.
12. Marks, T.A., Woodman, R.J., Geran, R.I., Billups, L.H. and Madison, R.M. Cancer Treat. Rep. 61, 1459-1470, 1977.
13. Schultz, R.M., Ruiz, P., Chirigos, M.A., Heine, U. and Nelson-Rees, W
14. Law, L.W., Dunn, T.B., Boyle, P.J. and Miller, J. J. Natl. Cancer Inst. 10, 179-192, 1949.
15. A generous gift of Dr. Margaret L. Kripke.
16. Schultz, R.M., Woods, W.A., Mohr, S.J. and Chirigos, M.A. Cancer Res. 36, 1641, 1976.
17. Fidler, I.J. Eur. J. Cancer 9, 223-227, 1973.
18. Liotta, L.A., Kleinerman, J. and Saidel, G.M. Cancer Res. 36, 889-894, 1976.
19. Hart, I.R., Talmadge, J.E. and Fidler, I.J. Cancer Res. 43, 400-402, 1983.
20. Fidler, I.J. Methods Cancer Res. 15, 399-439, 1978.
21. Click, R.E., Benck, L. and Alter, B.J. Cell Immunol. 3, 264-276, 1972.
22. Herber-Katz, E. and Click, R.E. Cell Immunol. 5, 410-418, 1972.
23. Peck, A.B. and Bach, F.H. J. Immunol. Methods 3, 147-164, 1973.
24. Swain, S.L. In: Selected Methods in Cellular Immunology, (Eds. B.B. Mishell and S.M. Shiigi), W.H. Freeman and Co., San Francisco, 1980.
25. Levin, J., Poore, T.E., Zauber, N.P., et al. N. Engl. J. Med. 283, 1313, 1970.
26. Wiltrout, R.H., Mathieson, B.J., Talmadge, J.E., Reynolds, C.W., Zhang, S-R., Herberman, R.B. and Ortaldo, J.R. J. Exp. Med. In Press.
27. Timonen, T. and Saksela, E. J. Immunol. Meth. 36:285, 1980.
28. Julius, M.H., Simpson E. and Herzenberg, L.A. Eur. J. Immunol. 3, 645, 1973.
29. Henry, C. (1980). Cell separation. In: B.B. Mishell and S.M. Shiigi (eds.) Selected Methods in Cellular Immunology. W.H. Freeman and Co., San Francisco.
30. Fidler, I.J., Raz, A., Fogler, W.E., Kirsh, R., Bugelski, P. and Poste, G. Cancer Res. 40:4460-4466, 1980.

31. Poste, G., Bucana, C., Raz, A., Bugelski, P., Kirsh, R. and Fidler, I.J. Cancer Res. 42:1412-1422, 1982.
32. Bach, F. and Hirschhorn, K. Science 143, 813, 1964.
33. Bach, F.H. and Voynow, N.K. Science 153, 545, 1966.
34. Bradley, L.M. In: (Eds. B.B. Mishell and S.M. Shiigi), Selected Methods in Cellular Immunology, W.H. Freeman and Co., San Francisco, 1980.
35. Brunner, K.T., Manel, J., Cerrottini, J.C. and Chapius, B. Immunology 14, 181, 1968.
36. Cerrottini, J.C., Enger, H.D., MacDonald, H.R. and Brunner, K.T. J. Exp. Med. 140, 703, 1974.
37. Gillis, S. and Smith, K.A. J. Exp. Med. 146, 468. 1977.
38. Henney, C.S. J. Immunol. 107, 1558, 1971.
39. Wagner, H. and Feldman, M. Cell. Immunology 3, 405, 1972.
40. Wunderlich, J.R. and Canty, T.G. Nature 228, 62, 1970.
41. Talmadge, J.E., Uithoven, K.A., Lenz, B.F. and Chirigos, M.A. Cancer Immunology Immunotherapy. In Press.
42. Talmadge, J.E., Oldham, R.K. and Fidler, I.J. JBRM 3:88-109, 1984.
43. Herberman, R.B., Nunn, M.E. and Lavrin, D.H. Int. J. Cancer 16, 216, 1975.
44. Kiessling, R., Klein, E. and Wigzell, H. Eur. J. Immunol. 5, 112, 1975.
45. Shiku, H., Bean, M.A., Old, L.J. and Oettegen, H.G. J. Natl. Cancer Inst. 54, 414, 1975.
46. Norbury, K.C. and Fidler, I.J. J. Immunol. Methods 7, 109, 1975.
47. Wiltrout, R.H., Taramelli, D. and Holden, H.T. J. Immunol. Methods 43, 319-331, 1981.
48. Talmadge, J.E., Lenz, B.F., Collins, M.S., Uithoven, K.A., Schneider, M.A., Adams, J.S., Pearson, J.W., Agee, W.J., Fox, R.E. and Oldham, R.K. Behring Inst. Mitt., 74:219-229, 1984.
49. Freireich, E.J., et al. Cancer Chemother. Rep. 50, 219-244, 1966.

3

PRECLINICAL EVALUATION OF INDIVIDUAL
BIOLOGICAL RESPONSE MODIFIERS

A.   Interferons
     (1)   Mouse interferon (β/α)
     (2)   Clone A recombinant human interferon
     (3)   Recombinant Human A/D BgL interferon
     (4)   Lymphoblastoid human interferon (Wellferon)
     (5)   Mouse gamma interferons

B.   Interferon Inducers
     (1)   MVE-2
     (2)   Poly ICLC

C.   T-Cell Immunoregulators
     (1)   Thymosin fraction 5
     (2)   Thymosin alpha-1
     (3)   Interleukin 2

D.   Natural Products And Extracts
     (1)   OK-432 (Picibanil)
     (2)   Lipopolysaccharide (LPS)
     (3)   Lentinan

E.   Synthetic Immunomodulators
     (1)   Nor-MDP
     (2)   FK-565
     (3)   Azimexon
     (4)   Bestatin
     (5)   Alkyl-lysophospholipids (ALP)
     (6)   N-137

F.   Specific Delivery of Therapeutic Agents to Macrophages
     by Liposomes

A: INTERFERONS

The interferons are a family of proteins and glycoproteins that are synthesized by cells in response to viral infection, antigenic challenge, and a variety of chemical inducers. Interferons can be produced by virtually all eucaryotic cells in response to a variety of stimuli and are capable of acting on homologous and heterologous cells with relative species specificity. The interferons that have been identified are divided into three major classes (alpha, beta, and gamma) according to their antigenic profiles, physiochemical characteristics, and inducing agents. Initially the interferons were categorized according to cell of origin, inductive stimulus, or physiochemical property such as acid lability. Leukocytes produce mainly α-IFN, fibroblasts mainly β-IFN, and T lymphocytes mainly γ-IFN. Interferon units are, at present, determined by a bioassay measuring antiviral activity. Interferons directly affect both malignant and normal cells by slowing their cycling time. This was initially demonstrated with the L-1210 lymphoma, whose growth in vivo as well as in vitro can be inhibited by interferon. Thus, the antiproliferative effects of interferon may account for some of the antitumor effects observed in vivo. In addition, immunomodulatory activities on virtually all of the cellular immune responses, distinct from antiproliferative and antiviral functions of the interferons, have been described. The interferons may also induce or regulate the expression of a variety of other lymphokines such as interleukin-2 (IL-2). Interferons appear to act directly on B cells depending on the relative timing of the exposure of the cells to antigen and interferon, and may either inhibit or stimulate pokeweed mitogen-induced immunoglobulin G (IgG) synthesis or antibody response to sheep red blood cells (SRBC). The T-cell response to a variety of antigens, including viruses and tumor cells may also be enhanced by interferon or be suppressed by the antiproliferative action of interferon or by the induction of suppressor cell activity.

Interferons also induce or augment the activity of non-antigen-specific effector cells such as macrophages and natural killer (NK) cells.

Whether interferon directly increases tumoricidal ability or primes the
monocytes or macrophages respond to a secondary signals such as lipopolysaccharide is controversial. Such is not the case with NK cells:
interferon can markedly increase activity <u>in vitro</u> and <u>in vivo</u> by recruit-
ment of pre-NK cells as well as by augmentation of NK-cell activity.

In summary, interferons may become an important class of biological
response modifiers (BRMs) for the treatment of cancer. Both the antiproliferative (on tumor cells) and immune augmentation (on macrophages
and NK cells) activities may play a role in the antitumor effects which
have already been observed in phase I and II clinical trials with this
class of BRMs.

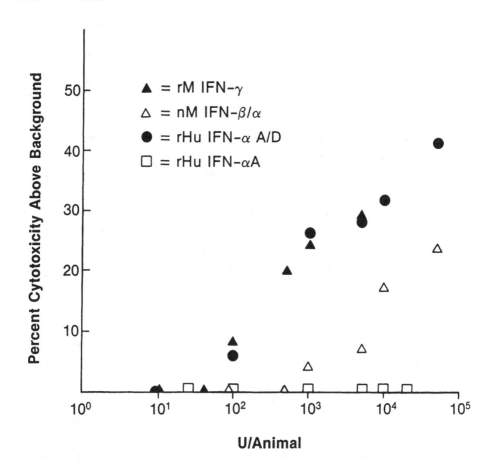

Reagents

Interferon	Species	Supplier
Recombinant αA	Human	Hoffmann LaRoche
Recombinant A/D BgL	Human	Hoffmann LaRoche
Natural α	Human	Burroughs Wellcome
Natural-B/α	Murine	Dr. Pauker's lab
Recombinant γ	Murine	Genentech

Augmentation of NK Cells (Dose Range Tested)

Interferon	In vitro dose (units/ml)	In vivo dose (units/animal)
rHu IFN-αA	1 - 20,000	25 - 100,000
rHu IFN-αA/D	1 - 25,000	1 - 200,000
nHu IFN-α	1 - 10,000	25 - 100,000
nM IFN-β/α	1 - 10,000	10 - 40,000
rM IFN-γ	0.01 - 1,000	10 - 50,000

The recombinant human (rHu) IFN-αA and the natural human (nHu) IFN-α were both unable to augment mouse NK cells either in vitro or in vivo due to species specificity. In contrast, the rHu IFN-α A/D was a potent augmenter of NK cells both in vitro and in vivo. The rHu IFN-α A/D is a molecular hybrid constructed by joining the N-terminal segment of rHu IFN-α A and with the C-terminal segment of rHu IFN-α D at the common BgL II site, amino acid position 63. The rHu IFN-α A/D has activity in vitro at doses as low as 100 units/ml and in vivo at 1,000 units per animal (20-g mouse). Maximal augmentation was observed at 500 units/ml in vitro and 10,000 units/ animal in vivo (Figure 1). Multiple injections of rHu IFN-α A/D induced an NK-cell hyporesponsive state in the spleens of mature mice that received 8 to 10 daily injections of 50,000 Units/ animal of rHu IFN-α A/D. The NK-cell hyporesponsive state was systemic, occurring not only in the spleens and peripheral blood lymphocytes of mice receiving multiple injections but also in the lungs and livers. Furthermore, the induction of an NK-cell hyporesponsive state was limited to adult mice that have maximal expression of NK cells and not mice with an age-associated reduction in NK-cell activity (3-wk-old mice or retired breeders >30 wk of age). Similarly, r murine (rM) IFN γ (50,000 units/animal) induced an NK-cell hyporesponsive state. However, multiple injections (qd) of low doses of interferon (rHu IFN-αA/D and rM IFN-γ) at 500 to 1,000 units/animal did not induce an NK-cell hyporesponsive state after 8 to 10 injections but rather augmented NK-cell activity to levels higher than those observed following a single injection. The rM IFN-γ also augmented murine NK cells in vitro following a 24-hr incubation and in vivo 24-96 hr following i.v. injection. The augmentation of NK-cell activity was observed in vitro at doses as low as 0.1 unit/ml and 50 units/animal in vivo, with maximal activity at 10 units/ml in vitro and 1,000 units/animal in vivo. In contrast, the nM IFN-β/α obtained from Dr. Pauker's laboratory (Philadelphia, PA) was less potent than either the rM IFN-γ or the rHu IFN αA/D. On a per unit basis (based on viral neutralization), the nM IFN-β/α required approximately ten fold higher levels of interferon to obtain similar levels of NK-cell augmentation both in vitro and in vivo. Thus, the nM IFN-β/α required 10 units/ml in vitro or 1,000 units/animal to significantly augment NK activity; maximal activation was observed with 50-100 units/ml in vitro or 10,000 units/animal in vivo. Figure 1 shows a comparison of the ability of these various IFNs to augment the splenic NK-cell activity in vivo with various doses of rHu IFNαA, rHu IFN-αA/D, rM IFN-γ, and nM IFN-β/α. It is apparent from this figure that rHu IFN-αA has no activity on mouse NK cells, while rHu IFN-αA/D and rM IFN-γ have a similar ability to augment NK-cell activity in vivo on a per unit basis, which is higher than that observed with the nM IFN-β/α.

Activation of Macrophages (Dose Range Tested)

Interferon	In vitro dose (units/ml)	In vivo dose (units/animal)
rHu IFNαA	1 - 10,000	1 - 100,000
rHu IFNαA/D	0.1 - 25,000	1 - 200,000
nHu IFNα	1 - 10,000	25 - 100,000
nM IFNβ/α	0.1 - 10,000	10 - 50,000
rM IFNγ	0.001 - 10,000	10 - 100,000

Similar to the studies on the augmentation of NK-cell activity, rHu IFN-αA and the nHu IFN-α were unable to stimulate macrophage cytotoxicity either in vitro or in vivo. However, the recombinant hybrid interferon (rHu IFN-αA/D) has immunomodulatory activity for murine macrophages. The rHu IFN-αA/D is able to activate murine macrophage tumoricidal activity both in vitro and in vivo. This material appears to directly activate the macrophages in the absence of detectable amounts of endotoxin; however, a second signal of 5 ng/ml lipopolysaccharide (LPS) greatly increased the tumoricidal activity when rHu IFN-αA/D was used to activate macrophage tumoricidal activity, as measured in an 18-hr ^{111}indium release assay. In contrast, the addition of LPS did not affect the activity of the rHu IFN-αA/D when examined in the 72-hr ^{125}I-IUdR assay using B16-BL6 as targets. In vitro macrophage tumoricidal activity was observed in the indium assays at doses as low as 50 units/ml and in the 72-hr ^{125}I-IUdR assay with doses as low as 1.0 units/ml. The rHu IFN-αA/D also activated alveolar macrophages and peritoneal macrophages in vivo following i.v. or i.p. injection, respectively, as assessed by the 72-hr ^{125}I-IUdR assay. The activation of murine macrophage tumoricidal activity in vivo required at least 500 units of rHu IFN-αA/D per animal, with maximal activity occurring at 10,000 units/animal.

The rM IFN-γ and nM IFN-β/α have also been found to activate macrophages in vitro and in vivo. The rM IFN-γ is a potent macrophage-activating agent, with activity as low as 0.01 units/ml and optimal activity at 10 units/ml as assessed in the ^{125}I-IUdR assay. The nM IFN-β/α is also capable of activating macrophages; however, it requires higher levels of interferon in vitro to activate with maximal activity at 50 units/ml. The rm IFN-γ is capable of activating macrophages in vivo, requiring 1,000 units/animal for maximum activation. When assessed in the 72-hr ^{125}I-IUdR or the 18-hr ^{111}indium assay, no second signal appears to be required for the activation of macrophages either in vitro or in vivo.

In summary, the rHu IFN-αA/D is capable of activating murine macrophages in vitro and in vivo with the requirement for a second signal apparently dependent on the assay of macrophage cytotoxicity utilized.

Furthermore, both nM IFN-β/α and rM IFN-γ are able to activate
macrophages in vitro and in vivo. In a direct comparison of macrophage
activation, based on virus neutralization titers, the rM IFN and rHu
IFN-αA/D appear to be approximately ten fold more active than the
nM IFN-β/α in the activation of macrophages in vitro.

T-Cells Immunomodulation (Dose Range Tested)

Interferon	In vitro dose (units/ml)	In vivo dose (units/animal)
rHu IFNαA	0.1 - 25,000	1 - 100,000
rHu IFNαA/D	0.1 - 25,000	1 - 100,000
nHu IFNα	0.1 - 25,000	1 - 100,000
nM IFNβ/α	0.1 - 20,000	
rM IFNγ	0.001 - 5,000	0.001 - 25,000

MIXED LYMPHOCYTE REACTION (MLR)

The addition of rHu IFN-αA or nHu IFN-α neither stimulated nor suppressed an allogeneic MLR. In contrast, the addition of rHu IFN-αA/D, rM
IFN-γ, or rM IFN-β/α suppressed an allogeneic MLR at doses ≥ 1,000
units/ml. However, these interferons did not stimulate or suppress the
background incorporation of tritiated thymidine into spleen cells cultured
in the absence of stimulator cells. Maximal suppression of the MLR occurred
with rHu IFN-α A/D at 10,000 units/ml, rM IFN-γ at 2500 units/ml, and nM
IFN-β/α at 10,000 units/ml.

ALLOGENEIC MIXED LYMPHOCYTE TUMOR RESPONSE-
CELL-MEDIATED CYTOTOXICITY (MLTR-CMC) ASSAY

In agreement with the results in the MLR, the addition of nHu IFN-α
or rHu IFN-αA to an allogeneic MLTR-CMC neither stimulated nor suppressed
the development of cytotoxic cells. However, the addition of rHu IFN-α
A/D, rM IFN-γ, or nM IFN-γ/α suppressed the development of cytotoxic
T cells during an allogeneic MLTR-CMC. Complete suppression of the development of cytotoxic T cells was observed following the addition of
20,000 units/ml of rHu IFN-α A/D; 10,000 units/ml of nM IFN- β/α, or 15 -
100 units/ml of rM IFN-γ.

Additional studies were undertaken with the rHu IFN-αA/D to examine whether or not this material induced suppressor T cells, which could depress the development of cytotoxic T cells in an optimal MLTR-CMC. In these studies, spleen cells in the presence or absence of stimulator cells were incubated in 25,000 units/ml of rHu IFN-α A/D. Following a 5-day coincubation, the cultured lymphocytes were washed extensively to remove any remaining rHu IFN-αA/D and added to an optimal (50:1, responser to simulator ratio) MLTR-CMC at a 10%, 1%, or 0.1% composition of the responders cells. In these studies, no evidence of suppressor cell activity was observed. Indeed, in the secondary cultures that received 10% or 1% of putative suppressor cells (lymphocytes cultured with stimulator cells and rHu IFN-α A/D), we observed increased development of cytotoxic effector cells. The secondary MLTR-CMC in the absence of stimulator cells that also received 10% or 1% putative suppressor cells also developed moderate levels of cytotoxic effector cells. This suggests that the rHu IFN-αA/D acted directly as an anti-proliferative agent and, after removal, allowed the expression of the cytotoxic T cells stimulated during the primary MLTR.

ADJUVANT ACTIVITY FOR THE DEVELOPMENT OF CYTOTOXIC T LYMPHOCYTES (CTL) AND FOR TUMOR CHALLENGE

Syngeneic tumor vaccines were injected i.d. in the presence or absence of various doses of the IFNs as adjuvants. Following immunization, spleen cells were removed and used as effector cells in a 18-hr radio-release assay using [75]selenium-radiolabeled tumor cells, or the mice were challenged with a tumor inoculum sufficient to induce tumors in 100% of the animals. In such studies, both rHu IFN-αA and nHu IFN-α had adjuvant activity for the development of CTLs and for the rejection of a tumor challenge. However, equal doses of human serum albumin, included as a carrier, had similar adjuvant-like activity and thus we could not demonstrate adjuvant activity specific for the IFN.

In contrast, rHu IFN-αA/D acted, in the absence of human serum albumin or any other exogenous proteinous material, as an adjuvant for the development of CTLs and to induce tumor rejection following tumor challenge. Optimal adjuvant activity was observed with 10,000 units of rHu IFN-αA/D per animal, with significant activity at 1,000 units of rHu IFN-αA/D per animal.

NONSPECIFIC IMMUNOPROPHYLAXIS

The i.v. injection of rHu IFN-αA/D, nM IFN-β/α or rM IFN-γ 48 hr prior to the i.v. challenge of UV-2237 mixed metastasis tumor cells significantly reduced the development of pulmonary tumor nodules. This occurred in a dose-dependent manner that directly paralleled the titration of the in vivo augmentation of NK-cell activity. In agreement with previous studies of NK activation, the i.v. injection of rHu IFN-αA or nHu IFN-α did not have any specific immunoprophylactic activity for the development of pulmonary tumor nodules.

IMMUNOTHERAPEUTIC PROPERTIES AGAINST EXPERIMENTAL AND SPONTANEOUS METASTASIS

The rHu IFN-αA and nHu IFN-α, in agreement with the immunomodulatory studies, had no therapeutic activity against either experimental metastases or spontaneous metastases of B16-BL6 at 100,000, 50,000, 10,000, and 1,000 units/animal when administered on a schedule of twice a week for 4 wk. In contrast, rHu IFN-αA/D had significant therapeutic activity against both spontaneous and experimental metastasis at 50,000 units/animal (twice a week for 4 wk) but not at 25,000, 10,000, or 1,000 units/ animal. The rM IFN-γ has had no therapeutic activity at 5,000, 1,000, 500, or 100 units/animal using the same schedule of treatment. Additional studies at higher doses of rM IFN-γ are needed to determine therapeutic activity.

B. INTERFERON INDUCERS

Interferon inducers include double-stranded RNA, certain chemicals, viruses, and various other microbial organisms. In this section, we will present data on maleic anhydride-divinyl ether (MVE-2) and poly ICLC from the Preclinical Screening Program.

MVE-2 (average molecular weight, 15,500) is a biological response modifier (BRM) that has been reported to stimulate the cytotoxic reactivity of NK cells and macrophages and to act as a T-cell adjuvant. The immunomodulation induced by MVE-2 has been variable when assessed in vitro and by in vivo therapeutic studies. Therapeutic activity in animal models has been reported, largely following i.p. injection directed against ascites tumors.

The synthetic, double-stranded nucleic acid polymer polyinosinic-polycytidylic acid (poly IC) is an effective inducer of interferon, activates NK cells and macrophages for cytotoxicity against tumor cells, and has prophylactic and therapeutic effects on viral infections and transplantable tumors in rodents. In addition, poly IC has been found to act as an immunoadjuvant, increasing humoral and cellular responses in selected systems. However, poly IC is a poor inducer of interferon in humans and nonhuman primates, perhaps because of serum ribonucleases that are capable of hydrolyzing poly IC. In 1975, Levy demonstrated that the complex of poly IC and poly-L-lysine, which was solubilized by the addition of carboxymethyl cellulose (poly ICLC), was an excellent interferon inducer in nonhuman primates. Poly ICLC induces moderate to high levels of serum interferon in rodents, nonhuman primates, and humans. Furthermore, poly ICLC has been found to have antiviral activity and to activate NK cells in nonhuman primates and humans. It has also been reported to augment NK-cell activity, delayed-type hypersensitivity responses, and lymphocytic blastogenesis. Poly ICLC has been given intravenously in several phase I/II clinical trials with the subsequent induction of serum interferon; a linear correlation between dose and peak interferon titer has been found.

Reagents

BRM	Supplier
MVE-2 Poly ICLC	Adria Laboratories Dr. Hilton Levy NIAID

Augmentation of Natural Killer Cells (Dose Range Tested)

BRM	In vitro dose	In vivo dose
MVE-2 Poly ICLC	6-100 µg/ml 0.001-100 µg/ml	3-50 mg/kg 0.0001-100 µg/animal

In vitro incubation of spleen cells with MVE-2 was unable to stimulate NK-cell activity. The i.v. injection of MVE-2 was capable of stimulating splenic NK-cell activity in vivo in a dose-dependent manner, slightly increasing NK-cell activity at 18 to 24 hr following i.v. injection (peak activity by 72 hr) with a return to near background levels by 7 days. The injection of 25 mg/kg MVE-2 induced detectable, but low (25 units/ml serum), serum IFN levels only at 3 days following i.v. injection.

In contrast to the increased NK-cell activity associated with a single injection of MVE-2, seven daily injections of MVE-2 resulted in splenic NK activity close to or below baseline levels. This hyporesponsiveness was observed after multiple i.v. or i.p. injections and was accompanied by splenomegaly. Hyporesponsiveness for NK augmentation was not observed after daily injections of poly IC. Daily injections of MVE-2 also depressed NK activity in peripheral blood lymphocytes, while the NK activity in the peritoneum, lungs, and liver was not suppressed but was higher than that seen at three days after a single injection of MVE-2.

Incubation of spleen cells with poly ICLC significantly augmented NK-cell activity in vitro. Incubation of poly ICLC with polymyxin B prior to addition to the spleen cells in vitro did not prevent the activation of NK cells by poly ICLC, indicating that, although poly ICLC reacts positively in the Limulus lysate assay and is also pyrogenic in vivo, the NK-augmenting properties are not attributable to contaminating LPS.

Poly ICLC also increased NK-cell activity following in vivo administration. When poly ICLC was administered either i.v. or i.p., peak activation occurred 24 to 48 hr following injection, with significant levels
of augmentation still observed 7 days but not 9 days following injection.
The s.c. injection or footpad injection of poly ICLC appeared to induce
NK-cell activation that was 2-3 days more prolonged than that observed
following i.v. or i.p. injection. A single i.v. injection of poly ICLC
was sufficient to activate NK cells in the spleen, peritoneal cavity,
peripheral blood, lungs, and liver.

The effect of multiple poly ICLC injections was examined to determine
its ability to maintain a sustained level of augmented NK-cell activity.
In this study, we found that the once-a-week or the twice-a-week injection
of poly ICLC was sufficient to maintain a high level of splenic NK-cell
activity and that more frequent injections did not induce further augmentation.

Poly ICLC was found to be a very effective inducer of interferon
activity. The injection of either 0.5 or 5 mg/kg of poly ICLC stimulated
increases in the level of interferon (IFN), with peak levels of IFN (6,000
units/ml serum) observed 24 hr following i.v. injection. Increased levels
of IFN were still observed 48 hr following injection of poly ICLC (0.5
mg/kg [100 units/serum] or 5 mg/kg [2,500 units/ml serum]). By 72 hr
after injection, no elevation in IFN titer was observed compared with
controls given saline injections.

Activation of Macrophages (Dose Range Tested)

BRM	In vitro Dose	In vivo Dose
MVE-2	6-400 µg/ml	1-50 mg/kg
Poly ICLC	0.0001-24 µg/ml	1-100 µg/kg

Incubation of C57BL/6N alveolar macrophages (AM) with MVE-2 rendered
them cytotoxic against syngeneic B16-BL6 melanoma cells in vitro. High
levels of cytotoxicity were observed, with concentrations of MVE-2 at
50 µg/ml or greater in the absence of detectable levels of endotoxin.
The tumor cell killing was not attributable to toxicity due to residual

MVE-2 since no cytotoxicity was seen in control wells without macrophages but incubated with MVE-2 for 24 hr.

The ability of MVE-2 to induce cytotoxic AM was also investigated following i.v. injection of MVE-2. AM activation was dose dependent and varied with the species studied, e.g., 25 mg/kg was required to activate the AM of C57BL/6N mice while a concentration of 5 mg/kg or greater activated the AM of F344 rats. The greatest activation of murine AM occurred at 50 mg/kg of MVE-2, a near lethal dose. It should be noted that even at near optimal levels, MVE-2 did not activate AM cytotoxicity to the same extent as did MTP-PE in MLV.

Macrophage activation was compartmentalized. The i.v. injection of MVE-2 activated only AM and not peritoneal macrophages (PM). Maximal activation occurred from 7 to 11 days following i.v. injection. In a parallel experiment, the i.p. injection of MVE-2 activated PM but not AM. The kinetics of macrophage activation following i.p. injection differed from that observed following i.v. injection. Peak activation occurred by 4 days following i.p. injection, but cytotoxicity was observed as early as 24 hr with i.v. treatment. Levels of AM-associated cytotoxicity following i.v. injection were considerably less than those observed with PM following i.p. injection.

The ability of poly ICLC to activate macrophages was studied by incubating C57BL/6N thioglycollate-elicited PEM with poly ICLC for 24 hr in vitro. Poly ICLC at levels of 1 µg/ml or greater did not activate macrophages to become cytotoxic in the 72-hr ^{125}I-IUdR assay. Indeed, poly ICLC at 10 µg/ml inhibited the slight spontaneous cytotoxicity associated with the PM in this assay. This high-dose inhibition of cytotoxicity by poly ICLC has been a consistent observation in the 72-hr assay. In contrast, doses of poly ICLC ranging from 0.1 to 0.0001 µg/ml were sufficient to induce significant macrophage activation, while doses of poly ICLC lower than 0.0001 µg/ml were incapable of activating macrophages.

Results similar to those obtained with the 72-hr assay using ^{125}I-IUdR-labeled adherent target cells were observed in macrophage-mediated cytotoxicity assays using ^{111}In-labeled nonadherent P815 mastocytoma cells in an 18-hr assay. Both studies resulted in similar levels of cytotoxicity but with a different dose titration for the activation of macrophages by poly ICLC. In the ^{111}In release assay, poly ICLC acti-

vated macrophages to become cytotoxic at doses from 0.5 to 10 µg/ml,
while lower levels of poly ICLC did not significantly stimulate cytotoxic
activity. The positive control LPS at both 10 and 1 µg/ml activated
macrophages to similar levels of cytotoxicity.

Poly ICLC activated PM or AM in vivo to become cytotoxic. Mice were
injected i.p. or i.v. respectively with poly ICLC and PM or AM were
obtained by lavage 24 hr later. Poly ICLC at 0.5 and 0.005 mg/kg significantly activated macrophage cytotoxicity in a 72-hr ^{125}I-IUdR release
assay; high doses (5 or 2.5 mg/kg) and low doses (below 0.005 mg/kg) of
poly ICLC did not activate the PM or AM. In agreement with the in vitro
18-hr ^{111}In assay, PM from mice injected with higher doses of poly
ICLC (> 0.5 mg/kg) were cytotoxic, while lower doses were not effective
in activating PM.

T-Cell Immunomodulation (Dose Range Tested)

BRM	In vitro Dose	In vivo Dose
MVE-2	0.5-100 µg/ml	1-25 mg/kg
Poly ICLC	0.01-100 µg/ml	5-100 µg/animal

MIXED LYMPHOCYTE REACTION (MLR)

MVE-2 was added to allogeneic MLR cultures, which were initiated at
a suboptimal stimulator:responder (S:R) ratio (1:10) in order to demonstra
maximum immunomodulation. The coculture of spleen cells in the presence
MVE-2 did not increase the proliferation in the cultures. Rather, at 50
and 100 µg/ml, MVE-2 significantly reduced the cpm incorporation into the
responding spleen cells. Modulation of alloantigen-driven T-cell proliferation responses by poly ICLC was studied in vitro using MLR cultures.
Poly ICLC significantly increased the allogeneic MLR when added at doses
of 1 and 5 µg/ml, with no significant enhancement at lower doses.
Higher doses of poly ICIC, i.e., 10 or 50 µg/ml, significantly reduced
the MLR response compared with the allogeneic cultures in control media.
Poly ICLC was unable to stimulate a blastogenic response in responder
cells cultured without stimulator cells.

ALLOGENEIC MIXED LYMPHOCYTE TUMOR RESPONSE CELL-MEDIATED CYTOTOXICITY
(MLTR-CMC) ASSAY.

MVE-2 was also tested in an allogeneic MLTR-CMC assay. The MLTR-CMC
assays were performed at a suboptimal S:R ratio (1:300) to permit the
demonstration of immunostimulation. At MVE-2 concentrations of 25 μg/ml
or greater, cytotoxicity was decreased below the level of that observed
with cultures in normal medium. This was due to toxicity since the cell
viability dropped from 72% to 20% with MVE-2. Since effector cell ratios
were calculated on the basis of equal numbers of viable cells, the lack
of cytotoxicity could not be attributable to insufficient levels of effector
cells. In addition, MVE-2 did not induce any "spontaneous" cytotoxic
effector cells such as might be associated with in vivo NK-cell activation.
Poly ICLC was also tested for the ability to stimulate the generation of
cytotoxic T effector cells during an MLTR-CMC. None of the doses of poly
ICLC examined significantly increased effector cell activity. At doses
above 10 μg/ml, significant loss of viability was observed in the spleen
cells cocultured with poly ICLC. Additionally, poly ICLC treatment did
not induce the development of any spontaneous cytotoxic effector cells,
as might be associated with in vitro NK-cell activation.

ADJUVANT ACTIVITY FOR THE DEVELOPMENT OF CYTOTOXIC T LYMPHOCYTES (CTL)
AND FOR TUMOR CHALLENGE

The immunoadjuvant activity of MVE-2 was assessed by examining its
effects on the in vivo stimulation of splenic cytotoxic T lymphocyte
(CTL) activity. Normal syngeneic mice were immunized by i.d. injection
of a suspension of lethally irradiated tumor cells obtained by the collagenase-DNAse dissociation of subcutaneous tumors. These mice received
a second vaccine 10 days later. Five days following the secondary immunization, spleen cells were removed and used as effector cells in an in
vitro assay of effector T-cell function. Mice immunized with tumor cells
alone had a slight increase in cytotoxic activity compared with spleen
cells from normal mice. However, the addition of MVE-2 to the vaccines
resulted in significantly increased levels of cytotoxic effector cells.
This adjuvant activity was consistently observed at 1 and 5 mg/kg of
MVE-2 but not at 25 mg/kg. The trypan blue viability of the tumor cells
in the vaccines admixed with MVE-2 at 25 mg/kg was less than 10% compared

with >90% at 1 and 5 mg/kg of MVE-2. Thus, the inability to act as an adjuvant at 25 mg/kg of MVE-2 was probably due to the loss of viable stimulator cells.

The immunoadjuvant potential of poly ICLC was assessed by examining its effect on the in vivo generation of splenic cytotoxic T-lymphocyte activity. Spleen cells from mice immunized with tumor cells alone gave a significant increase in specific cytotoxic activity compared with control spleen cells. Increased cytotoxicity was observed with vaccines admixed with poly ICLC, which had a dose-dependent effect, with 0.5 mg/kg augmenting the response while 5 mg/kg significantly inhibited the development of cytotoxic T lymphocytes. This decrease was due to poly-ICLC-associated toxicity for the tumor cells in the vaccine, which no longer excluded trypan blue and therefore, represented a loss of metabolically viable stimulator cells. Administration of poly ICLC alone, without tumor cells, did not induce increased levels of CTL compared with the mice receiving control (HBSS) vaccines.

In a second study, the effect of the route of adjuvant administration was examined. The BRM was delivered as an admixture with the tumor cell vaccine, or systemically by i.v. injection or by peritoneal injection to animals that also received i.d. vaccines. These studies revealed that poly ICLC was also effective as immune adjuvants when administered systemically in conjunction with an i.d. vaccine.

NONSPECIFIC IMMUNOPROPHYLAXIS

Three-week-old C3H mice received a single injection of MVE-2 and 48 h later were challenged with tumor cells by the i.v. injection. In this assay of immunoprophylaxis, MVE-2 significantly reduced the number of experimental metastases.

In one representative experiment in which splenic NK-cell activity was depressed (hyporesponsive state) by the daily injection of MVE-2 (8X), a decrease in lung colony formation was observed similar to that found in mice given a single injection of MVE-2. In both groups of mice receiving either a single or daily (8X) injection of MVE-2, a significant inhibition (Mann Whitney U test, $p <0.005$) in lung colony formation was observed compared with mice injected with HBSS. Further study revealed that the MVE-2 hyporesponsive state was not systemic but was associated with the spleen whereas pulmonary and hepatic NK cells remained augmented.

Poly ICLC significantly reduced the extent of experimental metastases as well as the number of mice that developed lung nodules. The pretreatment of mice with equal doses (total weight basis) of poly IC or poly ICLC induced similar resistance to the development of experimental metastases. The prophylaxis induced was dose-dependent: the highest doses of poly ICLC which were tested, 2.5 mg/kg or 5 mg/kg, were most effective in preventing the development of lung nodules. The lowest doses of poly ICLC (0.05 mg/kg) examined were less effective but still significantly reduced the median number of lung colonies produced by the i.v. injection of tumor cells ($p < 0.02$).

IMMUNOTHERAPEUTIC PROPERTIES AGAINST EXPERIMENTAL AND SPONTANEOUS METASTASIS

The therapeutic potential of MVE-2 was examined in mice bearing preexistent B16-BL6 lung nodules. In one study on the treatment of experimental metastases, therapy was initiated 72 hr following tumor induction with biweekly injections of MVE-2 for 3 wk. The mean survival time of untreated mice and mice given injections of HBSS was 41 and 43 days, respectively. Mice treated by the repeated i.v. injection of MLV incorporating MTP-PE demonstrated 60% survival on day 82, at which time they were necropsied and observed to be free of gross neoplastic disease. The treatment of mice with MVE-2 at 25 mg/kg prolonged the mean survival to 53 days. Therapeutic trials at 50 mg/kg proved to be toxic (weight loss, focal hepatic necrosis, and pulmonary thrombosis).

MVE-2 treatment of mice with preexistent spontaneous metastases whose primary footpad tumor was resected prior to therapy, did not reduce the number of mice with metastases. In contrast, the positive control, MLV incorporating MTP-PE, "cured" 50% of the tumor-bearing mice, thereby significantly reducing the median number of metastases.

In the experimental metastasis model, poly ICLC significantly reduced the number of experimental metastases in a dose-dependent manner and significantly prolonged the survival of mice bearing experimental B16-BL6 metastases. Poly ICLC significantly prolonged survival at 0.05 and 0.5 mg/kg as determined by the Kruskal-Wallis analysis values of (0.014 and 0.047, respectively), with 0.05 mg/kg poly ICLC having significantly better therapeutic benefit in this experiment than 0.5 mg/kg poly ICLC. Furthermore, treatment of animals with preexisting experimental metastases

with a dose of 0.05 mg/kg poly ICLC "cured" 30% of the animals. Syngenei
mice bearing UV-2237 Met-Mix pulmonary nodules were also treated with
poly ICLC starting either 2 or 8 days following tumor challenge. In this
study, poly ICLC at 1, 0.56, and 0.25 mg/kg was equally effective in
reducing the number of pulmonary metastases in the animals in which treatment was started 2 days following tumor challenge. In contrast, when
therapy was delayed until 8 days following tumor challenge, only poly
ICLC at 1 mg/kg was effective in significantly reducing the number of
pulmonary metastases. Thus, it appears that, although lower doses of
poly ICLC may be effective against minimal tumor burden, higher doses of
poly ICLC may be required in animals bearing extensive tumor burden.

The therapy of spontaneous metastases by the administration of poly
ICLC twice a week for 4 wk resulted in an immunotherapeutic response.
Mice that received HBSS injections developed a median of 10 spontaneous
metastases (90% incidence of metastases). However, mice treated with 2.5
mg/kg of poly ICLC had a median of 0 spontaneous metastases, with 70% of
the animals remaining tumor free at necropsy. Mice treated with 0.25 mg/k
of poly ICLC had a median of 3 pulmonary metastases, with 50% of the mice
tumor free. In another experiment, the control animals treated with HBSS
developed a median of 14 pulmonary metastases (100% incidence of metastase
and mice treated with poly ICLC at 1.25 mg/kg had a median of 0 pulmonary
metastases, with 55% of the mice remaining tumor free. Thus, poly ICLC ha
therapeutic efficacy not only against the limited tumor burden seen with
experimental metastases but also against well-established spontaneous
metastases in a tumor-compromised host.

SCHEDULING OF IMMUNOTHERAPY WITH POLY ICLC

Optimal scheduling of poly ICLC immunotherapy was investigated utili;
ing the experimental B16-BL6 metastases model in which therapy was initiat
3 days following tumor challenge. Significant prolongation of survival wa
observed when poly ICLC was given two, three, or five times per week. The
survival of mice treated with 1.25 mg/kg of poly ICLC administered twice
a week was significantly prolonged compared with those treated with 0.25
mg/kg (Cox's test, $p = 0.013$). However, on a three- or five-times-per-wee
schedule, both dosages gave similar results. Administration of poly ICLC
three or five times a week provided significantly better protection than

than twice-a-week administration (Cox's test, p = 0.0016). Because necrosis developed at the sites where multiple i.v. injections were given, injections were given i.v. following the first eight i.v. injections.

To determine whether the administration of poly ICLC for 4 wk was required or if a shorter schedule would be sufficient, poly ICLC was delivered on a suboptimal, twice-a-week schedule for 1, 2, 3, or 4 wk beginning 3 days following tumor challenge. No therapeutic efficacy was observed when mice were given poly ICLC twice a week for only 1 or 2 wk; however, at 0.5 mg/kg of poly ICLC, a significant prolongation of survival was observed when it was administered for 3 wk (p = 0.027; K/W analysis). When therapy was continued for 4 wk (both 0.5 and 2.5 mg/kg), it resulted in a significantly greater prolongation of survival compared to 3 weeks of adminiistration as determined by the K/W analysis (p = 0.0013 and 0.0007, respectively).

AUTOCHTHONOUS TUMOR MODELS

Poly ICLC has demonstrated therapeutic activity directed against UV-induced skin tumors and NMU induced mammary tumors. The optimal dose appears to be 0.25 mg/kg when administered i.v. on a three times per week schedule. The maximal therapeutic response requires the chronic adminis-tration of poly ICLC. Utilizing such a therapeutic protocol resulted in a significant reduction in tumor volume and prolongation of survival in both tumor models.

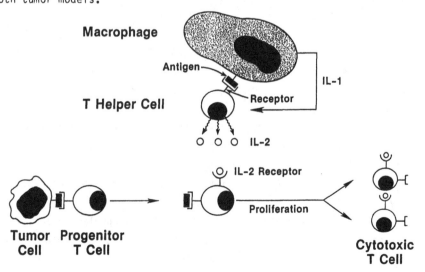

C: T-CELL IMMUNOREGULATORS

Thymosin fraction five (thymosin F5) is a complex thymic extract
containing a mixture of polypeptides with molecular weights ranging from
1,000 to 15,000 daltons. Thymosins play a role in the differentiation
and maturation of T lymphocytes and have immunopotentiating activities
that can restore some of the immunological responses in animals lacking
thymic function. The various peptides comprising thymosin F5 have different characteristics and may act individually or as a group at different sites and on different subsets of both pre-T cells and mature T-cell
populations.

Thymosin F5 has been reported to induce both helper and suppressor
cell activity. It appears that different lots of thymosin F5 are composed
of varying percentages of the individual polypeptides, which may account
for the disparate results amoung laboratories. However, the sequence of
several of the thymosin polypeptides is now known and at least one of them
(thymosin α1) has been synthesized and is available in large amounts.

Interleukin 2 (IL-2) is a glycoprotein of 15,400 daltons produced by
lymphocytes that have been stimulated by mitogens or antigens and was initially recognized due to its ability to maintain the in vitro proliferation of lymphocytes. Quiescent cytotoxic T lymphocyte (CTL) precursors
or undifferentiated T cells are insensitive to the stimulatory effect of
IL-2 and acquire a responsiveness to IL-2 following activation by antigens or mitogens. Activated CTL bind IL-2 and absorb the activity from
conditioned medium, while nonproliferating T cells do not. Thus, IL-2
may play a pivotal role in CTL proliferation and it appears that CTL
induction is dependent on IL-2 responsiveness.   The present working
hypothesis is that T-cell contact with specific antigen or mitogens up-
regulates IL-2 receptor expression, resulting in CTL precursors that are
suceptible to the stimulatory effect of IL-2. The IL-2 can be produced
by helper T cells in response to specific antigenic stimulation (Fig. 2).
Other regulatory molecules, such as interleukin 1, gamma interferon,
colony stimulating factors, or interleukin 3, have also been reported to
play a role in the development of active CTL in vitro. In addition to
these effects on T-lymphocyte differentiation and proliferation, IL-2
has been reported to activate natural killer (NK) cells (both in vivo and
in vitro) and/or lymphokine-activated killer (LAK) cells, although both

of these effector cells may be activated as a result of IL-2's stimulation
of the production of gamma interferon. Recent studies using IL-2 propagated CTL or NK cells have suggested that the concomitant injection of
these expanded lymphocytes and IL-2 may have some therapeutic properties.
However, no therapeutic efficacy by IL-2 alone has been demonstrated
against neoplastic disease.

Reagents

BRM	Species	Supplier
Thymosin F5	Bovine	Hoffmann LaRoche
Thymosin α1	Synthetic	Hoffmann LaRoche
Recombinant IL-2	Human	Biogen

Augmentation of NK Cells (Dose Range Tested)

BRM	In vitro dose	In vivo dose
Thymosin F5	0.001 - 500 μg/ml	1.0 - 1000 μg/animal
Thymosin α 1	0.0001 - 500 μg/ml	0.01 - 1000 μg/animal
rHu IL-2	0.001 - 50,000 units/ml	0.01 - 5x10^6 units/animal

Thymosin F5 and thymosin α1 did not augment NK-cell activity
either in vitro or in vivo. In contrast, the rHu IL-2 was a potent augmenting agent of NK-cell activity in vitro. In vitro incubation of
spleen cells with rHu IL-2 at doses of 10 units/ml or higher significantly augmented NK-cell activity, whereas lower doses of rHu IL-2 did
not augment NK-cell activity. Maximal augmentation of NK-cell activity
occurred with 1,000 units/ml of rHu IL-2. The admixture of rIL-2 with
polymyxin B (polymyxin B irreversibly binds to the lipid A moiety of
LPS, inhibiting its biological activity, including the augmentation of
NK-cell activity) prior to addition to the spleen cells in vitro did
not inhibit the NK-cell augmentation. Murine spleen cells needed to
be incubated with rHu IL-2 continuously for 24 hr to maximally augment
NK-cell activity. A brief incubation of spleen cells (10 min to 2
hr) in rHu IL-2 (200 units/ml) followed by an incubation in medium

for 24 hr did not significantly augment NK-cell activity. However, incubation of spleen cells for 7 to 16 hr with rHu IL-2 followed by incubation in medium for a total of 24 hr significantly augmented NK-cell activity but to a lesser extent than that observed following 24 hr of incubation. In contrast, incubation of very high levels of rHu IL-2 (2,000 units/ml) with spleen cells for only 2 hr was sufficient to augment NK-cell activity. Short incubations of spleen cells for 2 to 4 hr with rIL-2 at any dose, without a further period of incubation in media, did not augment NK-cell activity.

Recombinant human IL-2 also increased NK-cell activity following in vivo administration. The augmented NK-cell activity was sensitive to anti-asialo-GM1 antibody and complement but only sightly sensitive to anti-thy 1.2 antibody and complement. The i.p. administration of IL-2 stimulated peritoneal NK-cell activity but did not appreciably augment splenic NK-cell activity unless high doses (>100,000 units/ animal) were injected. The i.p. augmentation of peritoneal NK-cell activity required > 1,000 units of rIL-2 per animal, with maximal activity at approximately 50,000 units of rHu IL-2 per animal. Significant augmentation of peritoneal NK-cell activity was observed 24 to 96 hr after administration and returned to near background levels by 7 days. The i.v. injection of rIL-2 required > 100,000 units of IL-2 to significantly stimulate either splenic or peritoneal NK-cell activity, with maximal activity at approximately 1×10^6 units of rHu IL-2. The NK cells within the pulmonary or hepatic parenchyma are also augmented by rHu IL-2 following the i.v. injection of as little as 25,000 units of rHu IL-2.

Activation of Macrophages (Dose Range Tested)

BRM	In vitro dose	In vivo dose
Thymosin F5	0.01 - 500 µg/ml	1.0 - 1,000 µg/animal
Thymosin α 1	0.001 - 500 µg/ml	0.01 - 1,000 µg/animal
rHu IL-2	0.001 - 50,000 units/ml	0.01 - 1×10^6 units/animal

Similar to the studies on the augmentation of NK-cell activity by thymosin F5 and thymosin α1, these agents did not stimulate macrophage cytotoxicity either in vitro or in vivo. In contrast, the rHu IL-2 had immunomodulatory activity for murine macrophages both in vitro and in vivo. The rHu IL-2 activated murine macrophage tumoricidal activity in vitro following coincubation with thioglycollate elicited macrophage for 24 hr. The macrophage activation occurred in a dose-dependent manner, in the absence of any detectable endotoxin, and did not appear to be dependent on the presence of other lymphoid cells. Significant augmentation of macrophage tumoricidal activity was observed with 10 units/ml of rHu IL-2, with maximal activity occurring at approximately 1,000 units/ml of rIL-2. Purified peritoneal elicited macrophages, which were depleted of lymphocytes by pretreatment with anti-asialo-GM1 and anti-Thy 1.2 antibodies with complement and then further purified by adherence, could be activated with rHu IL-2 to become tumoricidal. Macrophage activation occurred in the presence of anti-gamma-interferon antiserum, which was sufficient to neutralize > 300 units of gamma interferon.

The rHu IL-2 was also able to activate PM following i.p. injection and AM following i.v. injection. Macrophage activation occurred with doses of IL-2 as low as 500 units/animal, with optimal activity occurring at 25,000 to 50,000 units of rHu IL-2 per animal. In all the studies of macrophage cytotoxicity to date (both in vitro and in vivo), the macrophage tumoricidal activity has been assessed using the 72-hr ^{125}I-IUdR assay with the adherent tumor target B16-BL6.

T-Cell Immune Modulation (Dose Range Tested)

BRM	In vitro dose	In vivo dose
Thymosin F5	0.01 - 500 µg/ml	1.0 - 2,500 µg/animal
Thymosin α 1	0.0001 - 500 µg/ml	0.01 - 1,250 µg/animal
rHu IL-2	0.001 - 50,000 units/ml	10.0 - 10,000 units/animal

MIXED LYMPHOCYTE REACTION (MLR)

The addition of thymosin F5 or thymosin α1 to an allogeneic MLR
stimulated the response in a dose-dependent manner. Optimal activity
was observed at 500 μg/ml, with significant activation noted at levels
as low as 10 μg/ml. Equidose concentrations by weight of thymosin F5
and thymosin α1 resulted in similar levels of MLR stimulation. Responder
cells cultured in the absence of stimulator cells also incorporated increased amounts of ^{3}H-thymidine in the presence of 100 or 500 μg/ml
of thymosin F5 or thymosin α1.

Maximal stimulation of the allogeneic MLR by rHu IL-2 was observed
at 500 units/ml, with far greater blastogenesis than that observed with
thymosin F5. A significant increase in the allogeneic MLR was observed
at levels of rHu IL-2 as low as 0.5 units/ml. The rHu IL-2 was also
found to be highly blastogenic when incubated with spleen cells alone,
i.e., in the absence of mitogen or alloantigen stimulation. Significant
blastogenesis was observed with levels of rIL-2 as low as 10 units/ml and
maximal blastogenesis at 500 to 1,000 units/ml of rHu IL-2. In most experiments, rHu IL-2 at concentrations greater than 250 units/ml induced
similar levels of ^{3}H-thymidine incorporation in both syngeneic and allogeneic cocultures. In addition, rHu IL-2 increased the blastogenic response of lymphocytes in response to suboptimal levels of Con A mitogenes

Additional studies were undertaken using human peripheral blood lymph
cytes to determine their response to rIL-2 in regard to a blastogenesis,
allogeneic MLR and stimulation of a suboptimal mitogen response. In all
analyses, the human peripheral blood lymphocytes had similar responses to
rHu IL-2 as those observed with the murine spleen cells. The minimal and
maximal concentration of rIL-2 were similar for the proliferation of both
the human lymphocytes and the murine lymphocytes.

Additional studies were undertaken to determine the nature of the
cells responding to rHu IL-2. Responder murine cells were treated with
anti-asialo-GM1 and complement, anti-Thy 1.2 and complement, or a complem
control prior to their incorporation into an MLR. Both antibody treatmen
reduced the normal allogeneic MLR response, while the pretreatment of the
responder cells with anti-asialo-GM1 antiserum significantly reduced the
blastogeneic response of responder cells in the presence of rHu IL-2.

However, the pretreatment of responder cells with anti-Thy 1.2 antiserum did not reduce the blastogeneic response of responder cells to the rHu IL-2. Nonetheless, in both assays (blastogenesis and allogeneic MLR) the incorporation of ^{3}H-thymidine was more depressed by pretreatment of cells with anti-asialo-GM1 in comparison with those treated with anti-Thy 1.2 antiserum. Human T cells and large granular lymphocytes (LGL), which are the morphological homolog of NK cells, were partially purified by Percoll density gradient and their ability to respond to the rHu IL-2 was examined. In these studies, the LGL responded in the absence of antigenic or mitogenic stimulus to rHu IL-2 in a dose-dependent manner and could be cultured in vitro in the presence of the rHu IL-2. In contrast, the partially purified unstimulated T cells had only a minimal response to rIL-2, which may be due to a small subpopulation of "activated" T cells.

ALLOGENEIC MIXED LYMPHOCYTE TUMOR RESPONSE-CELL-MEDIATED CYTOTOXICITY (MLTR-CMC) ASSAY

In agreement with the studies of the MLR, the addition of thymosin F5 or thymosin α1 to an allogeneic MLTR-CMC stimulated the development of specific cytotoxic T lymphocytes. Responder cells cultured in the absence of stimulator cells but with thymosin expressed an increased cytotoxic activity but at levels below that induced with stimulated cells. This nonspecific cytotoxicity occurred at 100 and 500 µg/ml of thymosin F5 or thymosin α1. Increased levels of specific cytotoxic T cells were induced in the presence of the thymosin at levels as low as 10 µg/ml, with maximal activity at 500 µg/ml. These effector cells were sensitive to anti-Thy 1.2 serum and complement lysis, anti Lyt-2.2 serum and complement lysis, but not anti-asialo-GM1 serum and complement lysis.

The addition of rHu IL-2 to allogeneic MLTR-CMC significantly induced cytotoxic effector cells when added to cocultures of stimulator cells and responder cells or responder cells cultured in the absence of stimulator cells. The increased effector cell activity by rHu IL-2 was independent of stimulator cells and was dose-dependent, with an optimal concentration of 500 to 1,000 units/ml. Significant augmentation of cytotoxic activity was observed in the presence of stimulator cells at 10 units of rHu IL-2 per milliliter, while significant augmentation of tumoricidal activity in the absence of stimulator cells was observed at 100 units/ml of rIL-2. The effector cells were sensitive to treatment with anti-Thy 1.2 antiserum and complement, anti-Lyt 2.2 serum and complement, but not anti-asialo-GM1 serum with complement. Thus, the effector cells induced in the presence or absence of stimulator cells have a classical cytotoxic T-cell phenotype.

ADJUVANT ACTIVITY FOR THE DEVELOPMENT OF CYTOTOXIC T LYMPHOCYTES (CTL) AND FOR TUMOR CHALLENGE

Mice immunized by the i.d. injection of a suspension of a suboptimal vaccine composed of lethally irradiated syngenic tumor cells in the presence of 25 mg/kg of thymosin F5 resulted in complete protection against tumor challenge. Lower doses of thymosin F5 (2.5 and 0.25 mg/kg) did not provide complete protection against tumor challenge but did act as an adjuvant that slowed tumor growth following challenge. The immune status was not due directly to thymosin F5 since the injection of thymosin F5 alone at a distant site did not prevent tumor outgrowth or reduce the tumor volume. The addition of thymosin F5 to a suboptimal syngeneic tumor vaccine at 125 and 12.5 mg/kg augmented the development of specific cytotoxic T lymphocytes, as assessed in vitro. Effector cells were tumor specific and required both vaccine and thymosin F5 for the induction of CTL activity. Similar results and dose levels were observed in studies utilizing thymosin α1.

Due to the increased activity of IL-2 following peritoneal injection, we utilized peritoneal vaccines of irradiated MBL-2 tumor cells for the development of cytotoxic T-lymphocyte vaccines, which were administered in conjunction with multiple doses of IL-2 (b.i.d. for 4 days). The incorporation of 100 units of IL-2 per injection stimulated the development of cytotoxic T lymphocytes. However, the injection of higher levels of IL-2, notably 10,000 units/animal, by the same schedule suppressed the development of any CTL induced with the vaccine alone. However, a single injection of IL-2 at 10,000 units/animal did not suppress the development of CTL activity. Therefore, IL-2 seems to have a bimodal activity such that high doses given several times suppress the development of cytotoxic T-lymphocyte activity, whereas lower doses augment the development of CTL activity. Optimal stimulation of CTL activity occurs at 100 units of IL-2/animal compared with a requirement of 20,000 to 50,000 units of IL-2 for optimal augmentation of peritoneal NK-cell activity.

NONSPECIFIC IMMUNOPROPHYLAXIS

The i.v. injection of thymosin F5 or thymosin α1 48 hr prior to the i.v. challenge of UV-2237 mixed metastasis tumor cells did not affect the development of pulmonary tumor nodules. The i.v. injection of rHu IL-2, in a dose-dependent manner, significantly reduced the development of pulmonary tumor nodules. Maximal activity was observed with 500,000 units of the rHu IL-2, with slight but significant activity being observed at 50,000 units of rHu IL-2 per animal.

IMMUNOTHERAPEUTIC PROPERTIES AGAINST EXPERIMENTAL AND SPONTANEOUS METASTASIS

The therapeutic potential of thymosin F5 and thymosin α1 were investigated using both experimental and spontaneous B16-BL6 metastasis therapy models. In the experimental metastasis therapy model, in which therapy was initiated 3 days following the i.v. injection of tumor cells, b.i.w. for 4 weeks, thymosin F5 and thymosin α1 significantly reduced the number of experimental metastasis. Optimal immunotherapeutic activity occurred at 5 to 25 mg/kg of thymosin F5, with significant activity at 0.5 mg/kg. A similar dose response was observed with thymosin α1, which also had optimal therapeutic activity at 25 mg/kg.

Treatment of spontaneous metastases with the thymosins in a twice weekly schedule for 4 weeks was also effective. Optimal activity was observed at 25 mg/kg with significant activity at 12.5 mg/kg of thymosin F5 or thymosin α1. Thymosin α1 also had significant therapeutic activity at 2.5 mg/kg, which was significantly less than that observed with 12.5 or 25 mg/kg of thymosin α1. Thus, both of the thymosins have therapeutic efficacy not only against a limited tumor burden (experimental metastases) but also against the established spontaneous metastases in a tumor-conditioned host.

The therapeutic efficacy of rHu IL-2 has been studied in a compartmentalized model consisting of MBL-2 tumor cells that were injected intraperitoneally and therapeutic protocols (t.i.w.) initiated 2 days following tumor challenge. In this study, rHu IL-2 i.p. at 10,000 units/animal caused a significant but slight prolongation of survival, whereas animals treated with 1,000 units or 100 units of rIL-2 had significantly better therapeutic survival than those treated with 10,000 units of IL-2. Therapeutic activity of rHu IL-2 has also been observed in the treatment of experimental B16-BL6 and M109 metastases. Optimal activity has been observed with the daily administration of 100 and 1000 units of rH IL-2. These results are similar to the dose-dependent efficacy observed in the development of cytotoxic T lymphocytes and do not parallel the augmentation of NK-cell activity.

D: NATURAL PRODUCTS AND EXTRACTS

PICIBANIL

Picibanil, or OK-432, is produced from cultures of a nonvirulent strain
of type 3, group A Streptococcus pyogenes. These cells are grown in
Bernheimer basal medium, and penicillin G is added for 30 min followed by
increased temperatures for 45 min. Picibanil is quantitated by KE units
(1 KE unit equals 0.1 mg dried [lyophilized] cells, which also includes
2.7 mg of medium salts [phosphate buffer, magnesium sulfate, and maltose]
and 2,700 units of penicillin G). Acute toxicity (death) is seen following i.v. injection of approximately 250 KE/kg for both rats and mice.
Chronic toxicity is experienced following i.v. injection of an amount
greater than 1 KE/mouse and greater than 2 KE/rat.

Picibanil has been reported to augment NK-cell activity, perhaps via
interferon induction, to activate macrophage tumoricidal activity, and to
act as an adjuvant for the development of cytotoxic T-lymphocyte activity.
It has also been reported to act as an immunostimulant for the development
of hematopoietic spleen colonies in irradiated mice.

Picibanil has been used in a number of clinical trials, most notably
in Japan, where a significant reduction in tumor burden as well as prolongation of survival has been reported. Perhaps the most impressive results
have been associated with i.p. administration of Picibanil in patients
with ovarian ascites, intraplural injection of Picibanil in patients with
pleural infusions, and transurethral injection into patients with bladder
carcinomas.

LENTINAN

Lentinan is obtained from the fruit body of Lentinus edodes, a popular
edible mushroom in Japan. Lentinan is a β-1, 3-glucan with an average
molecular weight of 500,000 daltons. Its repeating unit is composed of
5 β-1, 3-glucopyranoside linkages with 2 β-1, 6-glucopyranoside linked
branches.

Lentinan is reported to interact with macrophages, stimulate production
of IL-1, and augment the reactivity to MAF. Lentinan injected i.p. or
i.v. has not been reported to elevate phagocytic ability or to increase
the release of lysosomal enzymes. In contrast, it has been reported

that lentinan could induce cytotoxic peritoneal macrophages following
i.p. injection and i.v. injection. Lentinan does not induce interferon
production or stimulate the production of prostaglandins. In contrast,
the i.p. or i.v. injection of lentinan has been reported to stimulate
NK-cell activity, particularly in NK high responder C3H mice but not to
induce NK-cell activity in BALB/c mice. Lentinan has also been reported
to act as a T-cell adjuvant for tumor vaccines and to increase serum CSF.
It has been suggested that the adjuvant-like activity associated with
lentinan may be due to the augmented production of IL-1 by Ia-positive
immune regulatory macrophages.

Lentinan has been used extensively in phase I and phase II trials
in Japan. Most of these studies have been in patients with advanced or
recurrent gastric cancer. Similarly, lentinan has been reported to have
therapeutic activity in a variety of allogeneic and syngeneic tumors
models. Rose et al. (Cancer Res. 44:1368, 1984) reported that the most
effective therapeutic activity is observed with the Madison 109 tumor,
whereas the Meth-A fibrosarcoma has been reported to be nonresponsive
to lentinan. It should be noted that the both of these tumors are syngeneic to BALB/c mice, which are low NK responders.

In summary, lentinan is a well-characterized, purified, and relatively
nontoxic natural agent that has been reported to influence T-cell-mediated
cytotoxic immune responses, macrophage activation, and NK cell-mediated
responses. Both the NK-cell and macrophage augmentation appears to occur
in vivo but not in vitro with an adjuvant-like activity for T-cell respons
which may be associated with IL-1 production by macrophages and/or CSF
induction.

LIPOPOLYSACCHARIDE OR ENDOTOXIN

The outer cell wall of gram-negative bacteria is composed of a membrane biolayer. Projecting outward from this membrane are polysaccharides
that are linked to a lipid (lipid A) in the outer leaflet of the bilayer.
These lipopolysaccharides (LPS) are the endotoxins of gram-negative bacter
the toxic activity is associated with the lipid A, while the polysaccharic
are the "O" antigens of gram-negative bacteria.

Polymyxin B is a cationic polypeptide antibiotic that is effective
against most gram-negative bacteria. Polymyxin B binds irreversibly with

the lipid region of the LPS molecule therapy, reducing the biological activity toxicity of LPS.

LPS is a common contaminant of cell culture and immunological reagents. Sources of LPS include sera, media, growth factors, BRM's, autoclaved glassware, and other biological or chemical reagents. Furthermore, LPS is a potent immunomodulating compound that affects all aspects of the immune response and is a toxic compound in vivo.

LPS is a potent macrophage activating agent in vitro and in vivo as well as in the macrophage migration inhibition assay used to measure cell-mediated immunity. In addition, LPS-treated macrophages secrete large quantities of a wide variety of lysosomal enzymes. Exposure of macrophages either in vitro or in vivo to LPS increases phagocytosis and can also induce tumoricidal activity. Levels of LPS insufficient to induce tumoricidal activity can also act as a second signal for the induction of tumoricidal activity of "primed" macrophages. Augmented NK-cell activity can also be induced in vitro and in vivo by LPS. LPS has also been reported to act as a potent adjuvant and for T-cell-specific responses and is a potent B-cell mitogen. Endotoxin has also been reported to induce a variety of lymphokines, most notably tumor necrosis factor and IL-1.

Reagents

Agent	Supplier
Picibanil	Chugai, Japan
Lentinan	Ajinomoto, Japan
LPS	Difco, Michigan

Augmentation of NK Cells (Dose Range Tested)

Agent	In vitro dose	In vivo dose
Picibanil	0.000001 to 5 KE/ml	0.0001 to 5 KE/animal
Lentinan	0.1 to 500 µg/ml	0.1 to 50 mg/kg
LPS	0.000001 to 1 µg/ml	0.001 to 10 µg/animal

All three agents augmented NK cell activity in vivo, although lentinan did not augment NK activity in vitro. Picibanil was a potent NK-cell augmenting agent in vitro. In vitro augmenting activity was not observed at doses lower than 0.0001 KE/ml, with optimal activity being observed at 0.1 KE/ml. In over 10 assays of NK-cell augmentation in vitro, lentinan was unable to augment NK-cell activity in preparations such as those resulting from sodium hydroxide solubilization, and from homogenization-autoclaving and in preparations for clinical use. At 500 µg/ml, the lentinan was toxic to spleen cells following a 24-hr coincubation. Endotoxin is a potent NK-cell augmenting agent, with activity being observed in vitro at concentrations as low as 0.1 ng/ml. However, the threshold level of augmentation varies depending upon the age of the spleen cell donor. Optimal augmentation was seen at approximately 0.1 µg/ml.

In vivo augmentation of NK-cell activity was observed with doses of Picibanil as low as 0.1 KE/animal, with optimal augmentation occurring at 1 KE/animal. Slight interferon production was observed in animals at 24 hr following i.v. injection but not 72 hr following injection of Picibanil. The levels of interferons stimulated were dose-dependent, with the highest level obtained following the injection of 2 KE/animal. Maximal augmentation of NK activity occurred from 48 to 72 hr following injection and returned to background between day 7 and 9, depending upon the dose administered. There was a moderate compartmentalization of NK-cell augmentation such that the i.p. injection of Picibanil did not augment splenic NK-cell activity. Daily injections of Picibanil for 2 wk resulted in an NK-cell hyporesponsive state, in which the spleen cells did not have augmented cell activity. In contrast, their pulmonary and hepatic NK cells remained augmented. An injection of interferon or poly ICLC following 2 wk of daily administration of Picibanil and 24 hr prior to NK-cell analyses was sufficient to overcome the splenic NK-cell hyporesponsive state.

Lentinan was able to augment NK-cell activity in vivo following i.v. injection. The optimal dose of lentinan was greater than 10 mg/kg, with peak augmentation occurring 24 to 48 hr following injection. The augmentation of NK activity was short term, with a return to background level 5 days following a single injection. In contrast, endotoxin was a potent cell-augmenting agent, with optimal augmentation observed with 10 µg/animal although it was active at levels as low as 0.1 µg/animal.

In general, lentinan appeared to be a relatively poor NK-cell-augmenting agent (regardless of strain specificity), whereas Picibanil and LPS were both potent NK-cell-augmenting agents in vitro and in vivo. The augmentation of NK-cell activity by lentinan appeared to be independent of interferon stimulation since we were unable to demonstrate interferon induction at either 4 or 24 hr following the injection of 10 mg/kg of lentinan.

Activation of Macrophages (Dose Range Tested)

Agent	In vitro	In vivo
Picibanil	0.000001 to 5 KE/ml	0.0001 to 5 KE/ml
Lentinan	0.1 to 500 μg/ml	0.1 to 500 mg/kg
LPS	0.000001 to 50 μg/ml	0.001 to 10 μg/animal

Picibanil at concentrations from 0.5 to 0.0001 KE/ml acted as a potent macrophage activating agent in vitro or in vivo at dose greater then 0.2 KE/animal. Higher doses appeared to be toxic to the macrophages and were therefore inactive. In contrast, lentinan had no activating activity in vitro with $C_{57}BL/6$ mice at any of the doses examined. In these studies, we exclusively utilized a clinical preparation of lentinan that was endotoxin negative (< 0.03 ng/ml) by the Limulus amebocyte lysis assay. LPS was found to be a potent macrophage augmenting agent with activity as low as 10 ng/ml and optimal activity at approximately 100 ng/ ml. High doses of LPS (> 1 μg/ml) were inhibitory in the 72-hr ^{125}I-IUdR assay of macrophage tumoricidal activity. In contrast, in the 18-hr ^{111}In assay, minimal activity was observed at 0.5 μg/ml of LPS, with optimal activity at 5 μg/ml and no apparent inhibition of activity at doses as high as 50 μg/ml. Thus, there appears to be some difference in the assessment of macrophage activity between the two analyses: the ^{125}I-IUdR 72-hr assay appears to be much more sensitive to low doses of endotoxin, whereas the [111]indium assay is less sensitive but is not inhibited by high doses of LPS.

T-Cell Immunomodulation (Dose Range Tested)

Agents	In vitro	In vivo
Picibanil	0.0001 to 5 KE/ml	0.001 to 1 KE/animal
Lentinan	0.1 to 100 µg/ml	0.13 to 13 mg/kg
LPS	0.001 to 50 µg/ml	

MIXED LYMPHOCYTE REACTION (MLR)

The addition of Picibanil stimulated the proliferation of lymphocytes during an allogeneic mixed lymphocyte response (MLR). The optimal
concentration of Picibanil for the stimulation of the allogeneic MLR
was from 0.1 to 0.0001 KE/ml. The level of stimulation was decreased
at lower doses of Picibanil, while doses higher than 0.1 KE/ml inhibited
the incorporation of ^{3}H-thymidine during the allogeneic MLR.

Blastogensis was also observed in the lymphocyte cultures admixed
with 0.1 and 0.001 KE/ml of Picibanil. In contrast, lentinan did not
increase the proliferation of C_3H lymphocytes in the allogeneic MLR
nor did it increase the blastogenesis. At the highest dose of lentinan
examined (100 µg/ml), toxicity reduced the incorporation of ^{3}H-thy-
midine to background levels. LPS was also a potent stimulator of the
allogeneic MLR, with activity as low as 0.001 µg/ml and maximal activity
at 1 µg/ml. LPS was also blastogenic, with optimal activity at approximately 25 µg/ml, although significant augmentation of ^{3}H-thymidine
incorporation was observed at 1 µg/ml.

ALLOGENEIC MIXED LYMPHOCYTE TUMOR RESPONSE-CELL-MEDIATED
CYTOTOXICITY (MLTR-CMC) ASSAY

In agreement with the results in the MLR, the addition of Picibanil
to an allogeneic MLTR-CMC stimulated the development of specific cytotoxic effector cells. The coculture of spleen cells in the presence of
0.001 to 0.1 KE/ml of Picibanil increased the development of cytotoxic
effector cells in vitro. At concentrations above 0.05 to 0.1 KE/ml,
there was a significant reduction in the number of viable effector cells
following 5 days coculture, while lymphocytes cultured in Picibanil at
concentrations greater than 0.1 KE/ml were essentially nonviable following the 5-day coculture. In contrast to Picibanil, and in agreement
with the results in the MLR, lentinan was unable to stimulate the de-

the development of specific cytotoxic T-cells in tests with C3H spleen cells
in vitro. At the highest dose (100 µg/ml), there was a moderate reduction
in the viability in the the number of cells recovered from the cocultures.

The addition of LPS to allogeneic MLTR-CMC increased the development
of specific cytotoxic T cells in a dose-dependent manner with a bell-shaped
curve; at levels of LPS greater than 25 µg/ml, there was a reduction in
the development of cytotoxic effector cells. Similarly, levels of LPS
less than 0.001 µg/ml had no activity in stimulating specific cytotoxic
T cells. Maximal activity of LPS appeared to occur from 1 to 10 µg/ml.
The addition of Picibanil, lentinan, or LPS to lymphocytes cultured for 5
days in the absence of stimulator cells did not result in the augmentation
of any cytotoxic effector cell activity.

ADJUVANT ACTIVITY FOR THE DEVELOPMENT OF CYTOTOXIC T LYMPHOCYTES (CTL) AND FOR TUMOR CHALLENGE

Syngeneic tumor vaccines were injected i.d. in the presence or
absence of various doses of the immunomodulators as adjuvants. Following
immunization, spleen cells were removed and used as effector cells in an
18-hr assay using [75]selenium-labeled tumor cells and additional cohorts
of mice were challenged with a tumor inoculum sufficient to induce tumors
in 100% of the animals. In these studies, lentinan was unable to increase
CTL activity in C3H mice following its admixture in tumor vaccines. Furthermore, no specific prophylaxis was induced by lentinan in a adjuvant
setting. In contrast, when Picibanil was admixed with the suboptimal
tumor vaccine, it stimulated the development of specific cytotoxic T
lymphocytes. The optimal dose of Picibanil was 0.01 to 0.5 KE/animal,
while doses greater than 0.5 KE/animal were not effective. The injection
of Picibanil alone did not result in the development of specific or
nonspecific effector cells 10 days following the i.d. injection of the
compound. Specific immunoprophylaxis, using suboptimal vaccines admixed
with Picibanil as an adjuvant, reduced tumor incidence in all experiments.
The optimal vaccine dose was 0.002 to 0.05 KE/animal; higher or lower
doses were less efficacious.

Lentinan demonstrated a slight adjuvant activity in C3H and C57 BL6
mice with doses from 0.2 to 2 mg/kg. None of the challenged animals
rejected their tumor, but there was a reduction in the size of the tumors

and a delay in their induction following challenge.

NONSPECIFIC IMMUNOPROPHYLAXIS

The i.v. injection of Picibanil 24 or 48 hrs prior to the tumor cell challenge, at either 0.1 or 1 KE/animal, significantly reduced the occurrence of lung nodules in experimental animals compared with controls. In contrast, the prior injection of 5 KE/animal did not reduce the experiment metastases. Indeed, it appeared to increase the incidence of lung nodules which may be due to an artifact associated with the particulate nature of Picibinal and the effect of this compound on the integrity of the endothelial lining. Doses of lentinan from 1 to 10 mg/kg stimulated nonspecific effector activity in C_3H mice, which reduced the number of experimental metastases. The optimal dose was 10 mg/kg, although the lower doses significantly affected the number of lung colonies compared with the negative control.

IMMUNOTHERAPEUTIC PROPERTIES AGAINST EXPERIMENTAL AND SPONTANEOUS METASTA:

Picibinal demonstrated significant therapeutic activity in the treatment of both experimental and spontaneous metastases. In a direct comparison with poly ICLC, it was significantly less efficient, however, Picibina consistently resulted in the "cure" of approximately 40% of mice. Furthermore, in both the i.v. induced autochthonous skin tumor model and the NMU rat autochthonous mammary tumor model, Picibinal has demonstrated significant therapeutic activity. The biweekly injection of Picibinal for 4 wk followed by two weekly intralesional injections (5 KE/lesion) and maintenance therapy thereafter with biweekly injections of 1 KE/animal has resulted in the significant reduction in tumor burden and prolongation of survival. Optimal therapeutic activity with both transplantable tumors and autochthonous tumors, either mouse or rat, appears to require about 1 KE/animal.

In contrast to Picibinal, lentinan has demonstrated minimal therapeutic activity against transplantable B16 BL6 tumors. Nonetheless, most notably in the spontaneous metastasis model with this tumor, lentinan has shown significant reduction in the median number of spontaneous metastasis compared with saline controls. In comparison with the positive controls, (poly ICLC or MLV, MTP-PE) it was significantly less efficacious. In a study utilizing the Madison 109 lung carcinoma cell line, the biweekly i.v. injection of lentinan significantly delayed the outgrowth of intramuscular tumors when therapy was initiated when the tumor reached a 1-mm diameter and significantly prolonged their survival, but did not result in any tumor free mice. However, the positive control, poly ICLC also significantly reduced the growth of the primary tumor and rendered 50% of the animals tumor free. Thus, in agreement with the studies of others in mice, we found that lentinan has therapeutic activity that is relatively limited to the Madison 109 tumor and was not seen with B16-BL6. This difference may not be tumor associated but may be due to strain differences. Optimal therapeutic activity in all studies to date appears to be achieved by administration of approximately 25 to 50 mg/kg of lentinan.

E. SYNTHETIC IMMUNOMODULATORS

MURAMYL DIPEPTIDE

The peptidoglycan, muramyl dipeptide (MDP), or N-acetyl-muramyl-L-alanyl-D-isoglutamine, has the minimal adjuvant activity necessary to duplicate the immune adjuvant activity of Mycobacterium tuberculosis in Freund's complete adjuvant. Several analogs of MDP have also been reported to have adjuvant activity and enhance the host defense. The present studies utilized the analog nor-MDP (N-acetyl-nor-muramyl L-alanyl-D-isoglutamine).

MDP and many of its analogs enhance both the antibody response and cytotoxic T-cell response to antigens or tumor cells via adjuvant-like activity. MDP has also been reported to have a slight mitogenic activity for splenocytes as well as the ability to stimulate an allogeneic MLR. These analogs have also been shown to activate macrophages in vitro and in vivo, as measured by increased adherence and spreading, enzymatic secretion, production of prostaglandins, as well as tumoricidal activity. MDP is pyrogenic in rabbits, which is associated with the release of endogenous pyrogens by leukocytes. Indomethacin has been reported to inhibit the pyrogenic activity of MDP without affecting its immunoenhancing properties. MDP is rapidly eliminated: 30 min following i.v. injection, more than 50% of the material is recovered intact in the urine and 95% is recovered from the urine within 2 hr. These analogs have also been reported to have anti-neoplastic activity, particularly following intra-lesional injection. In addition, they appear to have therapeutic activity against a variety of infectious agents.

FK-565

The BRM, FK-565 ($C_{22}H_{38}N_4O_9$) is a synthetic derivative of FK-156 that was isolated from the fermentation broth of Streptomyces olivaceogrisus. This compound; N-[N^2-(heptanoyl-gamma-D-glutamyl)-muso-2 (L), 2' (D)-diamino-1-pinelmoyl]-D-alanine, is unique compared with MDP. It is devoid of the muramyl moiety: the heptanoyl group at the N-terminal end of the D-glutamic acid and the N-(meso-2,2'-diaminopimeloyl)-D-alanine residue at the gamma-C-terminal end of the D-glutamic acid are substituted.

FK-565 has been reported to have a slight mitogenic activity for murine spleen cells, and the ability to activate macrophage tumoricidal activity, and augment NK-cell activity both in vitro and in vivo. It has been reported to CSF production but not interferon production. FK-565 has therapeutic activity, including the suppression of tumor metastases in a model of nonspecific prophylaxis. In addition, FK-565 has been described to have prophylactic activity against infectious diseases and therapeutic activity against specific tumors when injected intralesionally.

AZIMEXON

Azimexon is a 2-cyansubstituted aziridine compound (2-[2-cyanaziridinyl-(1)]2-[2-carbamoylaziridinyl-(1)]-propane) This synthetic compound is slightly soluble in saline (10 mg/ml) with a short half-life in vitro of approximately 30 min. Azimexon is relatively nontoxic, with an acute toxicity in rodents of approximately 2 g/kg. This material has a serum half-life of approximately 6 hr, and minimal or no toxicity has been reported in clinical trials following injections of doses as high as 500 mg per patient.

Antitumor activity has been reported for azimexon in several syngeneic and allogeneic tumor models. A dose-response relationship has been reported for azimexon in patients with Lewis lung carcinoma, AKR leukemia, and K-B-23 fibrosarcoma, with maximal activity at 25 mg/kg. In all of these studies, the tumor was injected s.c. or i.v. and animals were treated b.i.w. for 3 or 4 wk starting 24 hr following tumor challenge. It has been suggested that the effector cells in these studies were a cytotoxic autoreactive cells (similar to NK cells), which are described as cytotoxic to both malignant and nonmalignant cells of syngeneic origin. High doses of azimexon (> 100 mg/kg) have been reported to stimulate T-suppressor cells and inhibit the activation of cytotoxic alloreactive cells. During in vitro studies, azimexon induced tumoristatic activity but not tumoricidal activity of macrophages. Azimexon has also been reported to augment the stimulation of lymphocytes by PHA or Con A, as indicated by increased ^{3}H-thymidine uptake, and to stimulate immunoglobulin secretion by B cells. The most noted effect of azimexon has been its myelostimulatory activity, perhaps due to the induction of granulocyte-macrophage colony stimulating factor.

In animals immunosuppressed by cytotoxic agents or radiation, azimexon has been reported to enhance the recovery from leukopenia and low T-cell activity. However, no significant reversal of chemotherapy-induced myelosuppression has been demonstrated clinically.

BESTATIN

Bestatin is a low molecular weight factor originally isolated from culture supernatants of Streptomyces olivoreticuli, which is a potent competitive inhibitor for aminopeptidase B and leucine aminopeptidase. This enzyme inhibitor, bestatin ([2S, 3R-3-amino-2-hydroxy-4-phenyl, butanoyl]-L-leucine), has been reported to have both immunomodulatory and immunotherapeutic properties. Bestatin has been shown to increase proliferation of T lymphocytes, perhaps by the induction of macrophage-produced monokines. Bestatin has also been reported to increase the activity of DNA polymerase alpha and terminal deoxynucleotide transferase in T cells, increase DTH responses, act as an adjuvant for plaque forming cells, augment macrophage-mediated cytostasis and cytotoxicity, as well as augment the production of colony forming activity. In addition, prophylactic studies with bestatin have demonstrated protection against bacterial challenges. Bestatin has also been reported to inhibit the growth of several syngeneic tumors, including myeloid leukemia and colon carcinoma. Bestatin has been examined in several phase I trials and was found to induce minimal toxicity even with doses as high as 800 mg administered daily. In these clinical trials, bestatin was reported to increase the DTH, augment immunoglobulin production, augment NK cell activity, and increase the percentage of E-rosettes in immunodepressed patients.

ALKYL-LYSOPHOSPHOLIPIDS

Alkyl-lysophospholipid (ALP) (Et-C_{18}-OCH$_3$ [racemic 1-ocetadecyl-2-methoxyglycero-3-phosphocholine]) is a synthetic analogue of the natural compound 2-lysophosphatidylcholine. ALP is directly cytotoxic to tumor cells in vitro and presumably in vivo. It also activates macrophages to become tumoricidal following in vitro coincubation and in vivo following i.p. injection.

ALP has been reported to have prophylactic potential when injected prior to tumor challenge. In addition, the chronic administration of ALP prolonged the survival of animals bearing subcutaneous tumors and, if combined with resection, to reduce the development of metastases in animals with Lewis lung carcinoma. In summary, the alkyl-lysophospholipids are toxic, have macrophage activating properties, and appear to have both prophylactic and therapeutic activities in vivo.

N-137

N-137 is a bifunctional polymer of small molecule weight (MW=800) consisting of alternating charged groups on a carbon backbone. N-137 is a copolymer of ethylene and maleic anhydride which has been reported to have adjuvant activity for both B cells and T cells. N-137 also has been reported to have some therapeutic activity in tumor-bearing animals as well as activity against metastases when treatment was initiated following resection of a primary bladder carcinoma. In addition, there is evidence of a direct growth inhibitory effect by N-137 on both murine and human tumors.

Reagents

Agent	Supplier
Muramyl dipeptide	Ciba Geigy
FK-565	Fujisawa Pharm
Azimexon	Boehringer Mannheim
Bestatin	Dr. Umezawa, Microbial Research Foundation, Toyoko
Alkyl-lysophospholipid	Dr. Berdel, Munich, Germany
N-137	Monsanto, St. Louis

Augmentation of NK Cells (Dose Range Tested)

Agent	In Vitro	In Vivo
Muramyl dipeptide	3-300 µg/ml	0.15-100 mg/kg
FK-565	0.0001-100 µg/ml	2.5-50 mg/kg
Azimexon	0.01-1,600 µg/ml	6-500 mg/kg
Bestatin	0.01-500 µg/ml	0.1-500 mg/kg
Alkyl-lysophospholipids	0.00001-1 µg/ml	0.5 mg/kg-50 mg/kg
N-137	1-500 µg/ml	0.5-50 mg/kg

Nor-MDP, azimexon, alkyl-lysophospholipids, bestatin, and N-137
were all unable to augment NK cell activity, either in vitro or in vivo.
In contrast, FK-565 was a potent augmenting agent for NK-cell activity.
In vitro augmentation of NK-cell activity by FK-565 occurred at extremely
low levels of FK-565, with significant augmentation induced at 0.001 μg/
ml and peak augmentation occurring at approximately 1 μg/ml. NK-cell
augmentation by FK-565 was not observed 24 hr following i.v. or i.p. injection of FK-565. However, at 3 or 5 days following i.v. injection of
FK-565, augmented NK-cell activity was observed. The NK-cell augmentation
returned to background levels 9 days following i.v. injection. Maximal
augmentation occurred at 2.5 mg/kg, and the minimum dose capable of augmenting NK activity was 0.5 mg/kg.

Activation of Macrophages (Dose Range Tested)

Agent	In vitro	In vivo
Muramyl dipeptide	3-1,000 μg/ml	0.15-200 mg/kg
FK-565	0.001-100 μg/ml	0.05-5 mg/kg
Azimexon	6-100 μg/ml	6-100 mg/kg
Bestatin	0.0001-500 μg/ml	0.005-5 mg/kg
Alkyl-lysophospholipids	0.000001-500 μg/ml	0.01-10 mg/kg
N-137	1-100 μg/ml	1.0-100 mg/kg

Azimexon was unable to augment macrophage tumoricidal activity
either in vitro or in vivo. Nor-MDP, however, was a potent activator
of macrophage cytotoxicity in vitro, with activation occurring at
100 μg/ml and maximal activity at 1,000 μg/ml. However, Nor-MDP
was less active in vivo: alveolar macrophage activation following
i.v. injection required doses greater than 50 mg/kg. This presumably
is due to the rapid in vivo excretion of MDP. FK-565 was also a potent
macrophage activating agent, with stimulatory effects seen with 0.01 to
500 μg/ml. The optimal dose appeared to be 10 to 50 μg/ml, with
the higher doses somewhat less active. FK-565 was also capable of
augmenting alveolar macrophages following i.v. injection or peritoneal
macrophages following i.p. injection, with maximal activity at 0.75 to

5.0 mg/kg, although doses as low as 0.1 mg/kg also significantly activated macrophage tumoricidal properties. In comparison with Nor-MDP, FK-565 demonstrated macrophage activation both in vitro and in vivo at much lower doses. Bestatin was also capable of augmenting macrophage tumoricidal properties both in vitro and in vivo. It augmented macrophage-mediated tumoricidal ability in vitro at doses from 0.1 through 500 µg/ml, with optimal effects of approximately 10 to 50 µg/ml. Bestatin was also a potent in vivo macrophage augmenting agent, with activity as low as 0.05 mg/kg and optimal activity at approximately 1 mg/kg. Macrophage augmentation was somewhat assay dependent, with optimal activation occurring in the 72-hr ^{125}I-IUdR assay and minimal activity in an 18-hr ^{111}In release assay. The addition of nonactivating levels of LPS (5 ng/ml) increased the macrophage activity primed by bestatin. ALP was also capable of activating macrophage cytotoxicity in vitro at doses from 0.0001 to 10 µg/ml, as determined using the 72-hr ^{125}I-IUdR assay but not the 18-hr ^{111}indium assay. ALP at concentrations greater than 20 µg/ml was toxic to both macrophages and target cells. This material is extremely "sticky" and appropriate control wells are required in assays of cytotoxicity. ALP was also capable of activating macrophages in vivo following i.v. injection, with optimal activation of alveolar macrophages at 0.05 to 1 mg/kg. N-137 was unable to activate murine macrophages in vitro in either the 72-hr ^{125}I-IUdR assay or the 18-hr ^{111}In assay. In contrast, alveolar macrophages and peritoneal macrophages were activated following i.v. or i.p. injection, respectively. Optimal activity was observed at 1 to 5 mg/kg.

T-Cell Immunomodulation (Dose Range Tested)

Agent	In vitro	In vivo
Muramyl dipeptide	1-300 µg/ml	1-75 mg/kg
FK-565	0.0001-100 µg/ml	0.025-15 mg/kg
Azimexon	0.1-100 µg/ml	1-100 mg/kg
Bestatin	0.01-100 µg/ml	0.025-25 mg/kg
Alkyl-lysophospholipids	0.0001-1 µg/ml	0.215-250 µg/kg
N-137	0.1 µg/ml-1 mg/ml	0.5-1,000 mg/kg

MIXED LYMPHOCYTE REACTION (MLR)

Both Nor-MDP and FK-565 stimulated a suboptimal allogeneic mixed lympocyte response. The optimal concentration of Nor-MDP was from 30 to 100 µg/ml, whereas optimal stimulation with FK-565 occurred at 0.1 µg/ml. Nor-MDP was nonblastogenic to spleen cells cultured alone while FK-565 was slightly blastogenic from 0.01 to 1 µg/ml. Significant depression of allogeneic stimulation was observed with 100 µg/ml of FK-565. Azimexon increased the allogeneic MLR in approximately 50% of the assays, with maximum activity at 10 to 25 µg/ml. Higher doses of azimexon (50 to 100 µg/ml) decreased ^{3}H-thymidine incorporation. No blastogenic activity was associated with the addition of azimexon. Bestatin was also capable of increasing an allogeneic MLR, with optimal stimulation from 1 to 10 µg/ml. Additionally, a slight blastogenesis was observed when responder lymphocytes were cultured alone in the presence of 10 µg/ml bestatin. The allogeneic MLR stimulation was depressed somewhat by 100 µg/ml of bestatin, suggestive of a slight toxicity. ALP was capable of increasing the allogeneic MLR, with optimal activity from 0.001 to 0.1 µg/ml. Concentrations of ALP greater than 1 µg/ml were toxic to the lymphocytes and severely depressed the incorporation of ^{3}H-thymidine. No blastogenesis was observed at any concentration tested. N-137 was not blastogenic, and did not increase an allogeneic MLR.

ALLOGENEIC MIXED LYMPHOCYTE TUMOR RESPONSE-CELL-MEDIATED CYTOTOXICITY (MLTR-CMC) ASSAY

In agreement with the results of the mixed lymphocyte response, the addition of Nor-MDP and FK-565 to an allogeneic MLTR-CMC stimulated the development of specific cytotoxic T cells. The optimal dose of Nor-MDP was 10 to 30 µg/ml, whereas the optimal dose of FK-565 was 0.1 to 1.0 µg/ml. Significant augmentation of cytotoxic T lymphocytes occurred at levels of FK-565 as low as 0.001 µg/ml. There was no tendency for decreased cytotoxic T-cell activity at doses of FK-565 as high as 100 µg/ml In both cases (Nor-MDP and FK-565), there was no induction of nonspecific effector cells in cultures of responder cells admixed with the agent alone. The addition of azimexon, bestatin, ALP, or N-137 did not stimulate the development of cytotoxic T cells in a suboptimal allogeneic MLTR-CMC. Concentrations of ALP greater than 1.0 µg/ml were signifi-

cantly toxic, reducing the number of viable spleen cells following co-
culture. Thus, in contrast to their ability to stimulate an allogeneic
MLR, these agents were unable to increase the development of cytotoxic
T lymphocytes following coculture in an allogeneic MLTR-CMC.

ADJUVANT ACTIVITY FOR THE DEVELOPMENT OF CYTOTOXIC T LYMPHOCYTES (CTL)
AND FOR TUMOR CHALLENGE

Syngeneic tumor vaccines were injected i.d. in the presence or
absence of various doses of the BRM as adjuvants. Following immunization,
spleen cells were removed and used as effector cells in an 18-hr radioisotope release assay using ^{75}selenium radio-labeled tumor cells as
targets. In addition, groups of immunized mice were challenged with a
tumor inoculum sufficient to induce tumors in 100% of the animals. The
admixture of Nor-MDP or FK-565 with a suboptimal tumor vaccine resulted
in the development of specific cytotoxic T lymphocytes as well as the
rejection of tumor transplants. The optimal dose of Nor-MDP was 75
mg/kg, while lower doses were not effective as adjuvants. In contrast,
the optimal dose of FK-565 was 0.25 to 1 mg/kg, with higher doses somewhat
less efficacious as an adjuvant. The injection of either BRM alone did
not result in the activation of polyclonal cytotoxic effector cells.
Additional studies revealed that the concomitant injection of an i.d.
tumor vaccine with the i.v. injection of FK-565 also resulted in the
stimulation of cytotoxic T lymphocytes.

As discussed in Ch 3, chronic UV irradiation of animals results
in skin tumors that are in general highly antigeneic. These tumors
differ from those induced by chemical carcinogens, such that the majority
are rejected following transplantation to normal syngeneic mice but
grow progressively in immunosuppressed recipients or in mice that have
received chronic, subtumorigenic UV irradiation. Prior to the development of primary skin tumors, mice that have been UV irradiated lose
their ability to reject transplants of regressor UV-induced tumors by a
mechanism that involves T-cell-mediated immmunosuppression. This immunological hyporesponsiveness extends to all syngeneic UV-induced tumors
but not to other non-UV-induced tumors. The immunological aspect of
this systemic alteration can be adoptively transferred with lymphoid
cells from UV-irradiated mice into lethally irradiated normal recipients.

The suppressors cells express membrane-associated Thy-1 antigens and are radiation sensitive.

Mice that have received subtumorigenic UV irradiation and have suppressor T cells are unable to respond to tumor vaccines of UV-induced tumors. Regardless of the nature of the tumor vaccine, such animals will not reject an appropriate tumor challenge. However, if Nor-MDP or FK-565 is admixed as an adjuvant, a moderate degree of specific protection is induced. The addition of Nor-MDP as an adjuvant provides protection to approximately 30% of the animals following tumor challenge when it is admixed at 100 mg/kg. In contrast, the addition of FK-565 as an adjuvant at 10 mg/kg resulted in complete protection against tumor challenge, suggesting that the use of FK-565 as an adjuvant might overcome the presence of suppressor T cells, resulting in the development of specific cytotoxic effector cells that can cause the rejection of tumor challenge.

Azimexon also acted as an adjuvant for suboptimal tumor vaccines in normal mice, with an optimal activity at 25 mg/kg. Similarly, bestatin, ALP, and N-137 acted as adjuvants following admixture with suboptimal tumor vaccine. Optimal doses for tumor vaccines were 1 through 25 mg/kg, 0.5 to 10 µg/kg, and 5 to 50 mg/kg, respectively. In all cases, the injection of the BRM alone, in the absence of the tumor vaccine, did not result in the development of nonspecific effector cells nor did it result in any protection against tumor challenge. In every case, a suboptimal tumor vaccine with a positive immunoadjuvant also resulted in the rejection of tumor challenge as well as the development of cytotoxic T lymphocytes.

NONSPECIFIC IMMUNOPROPHYLAXIS

In agreement with the inability of in vivo injections of these BRMs to augment NK cell activity, the i.v. injection of Nor-MDP, azimexon, ALP, bestatin, and N-137 did not reduce the development of pulmonary tumor nodules. However, again in agreement with in vivo NK augmentation studies, the injection of FK-565 72 hr prior to the i.v. challenge with tumor cells significantly reduced the development of pulmonary nodules. This occurred in a dose-dependent manner that directly paralleled the titration of the in vivo augmentation of NK-cell activity.

IMMUNOTHERAPEUTIC PROPERTIES AGAINST EXPERIMENTAL AND SPONTANEOUS METASTASES

The biweekly administration of Nor-MDP at 15 mg/kg but not lower doses resulted in a 40% long-term survival of animals bearing experimental B16-BL6 pulmonary metastases. Similarly, the treatment of animals with spontaneous B16-BL6 metastases with 50 mg/kg (administered three times per week) also resulted in significant therapeutic benefit, although the treatment of animals either once or twice a week was not effective. In contrast, the treatment of mice with experimental B16-BL6 metastases with 25 mg/kg of FK-565, injected either twice a week or three times per week, significantly reduced the median number of metastases, prolonged survival and gave a 60% "cure". Therapeutic activity was also observed with 10 and 2.5 mg/kg of FK-565. Higher levels of FK-565 (50 or 75 mg/kg) were less efficacious than the optimal dose of 25 mg/kg. There did not appear to be any therapeutic advantage to the administration of FK-565 three times per week compared with two times per week. Treatment of mice with spontaneous B16-BL6 metastases following the resection of the primary footpad tumor using FK-565 at 25 and 50 mg/kg resulted in therapeutic activity. However, no therapeutic activity was observed at 5 mg/kg of FK-565. Treatment of mice with experimental metastases using azimexon at 5 to 100 mg/kg did not reduce the median number of metastases or prolong the survival of the mice. However, the treatment of animals bearing spontaneous pulmonary metastases following the resection of a primary tumor (treatment 3 times per week for 4 wk) reduced the median number of spontaneous metastases and "cured" 30% of the animals. Bestatin also demonstrated significant therapeutic activity for both experimental and spontaneous metastases. In these studies, bestatin doses of 50 or 100 mg/kg delivered twice a week were required for therapeutic activity. Lower doses of bestatin (25 mg/kg) had no therapeutic activity. Similarly, 50 mg/kg or 100 mg/kg of bestatin injected twice a week for 4 wk following the resection of a primary footpad tumor significantly prolonged the survival of animals and reduced the median number of spontaneous metastases. In contrast, ALP and N-137 had appreciably less therapeutic activity: the treatment of animals with ALP at 15 mg/kg slightly prolonged the survival of animals with experimental metastases, although it did not prolong the survival nor reduce the secondary tumor burden in animals with spontaneous metastases. N-137 also had some slight therapeutic activity against experimental metastases and reduced the median number of metastases at 0.25 and 2.5 mg/kg. In the treatment of spontaneous metastases, N-137 did reduce the median number of spontaneous metastases when administered at 10 mg/kg, although higher doses had no therapeutic activity. In the studies with ALP and N-137, the positive controls, thymosin F5, poly ICLC, and liposomes incorporating MTP-PE, had significantly better therapeutic activity (in terms of reduction of metastasis and prolongation of survival). In contrast, the treatment protocols using Nor-MDP, FK-565, and bestatin therapeutic activity had similar or better therapeutic activity compared with the positive controls.

F: SPECIFIC DELIVERY OF THERAPEUTIC AGENTS TO MACROPHAGES BY LIPOSOMES

Liposomes are lipid vesicles consisting of one or several concentric lipid bilayers surrounding an internalized aqueous space. They can be prepared from a wide range of phospholipids, either in pure form, or in combination with other amphipathic molecules such as sterols, long chain bases or acids, or integral membrane proteins. Liposomes can be constructed to meet a diversity of experimental requirements by altering such characteristics as surface charge, permeability to ions, and the physical state of the lipids. Liposomes of widely differing size can be prepared, ranging from large (0.5-10 μ diameter) multilamellar (MLV) or unilammellar liposomes to small (~300 Å diameter) unilamellar liposomes (SUV). A wide range of biologically-active molecules and macromolecules have been incorporated into liposomes either in association with the liposome membrane or encapsulated within the aqueous space(s) of the liposome interior. The potential value of liposomes as carriers for improving drug delivery _in vivo_ has attracted considerable attention in the last few years in large part because it was thought possible to "target" these structures to specific cell types, including tumor cells. Successful targeting of this kind has not been achieved. Consequently, even if liposomes with appropriate "cell recognition molecules" could be constructed, the anatomic barrier imposed by the vascular tree would frustrate their access to "target" cells in extravascular tissue. Studies on the distribution of liposomes injected i.v. have shown that they localize predominantly in organs with high reticuloendothelial (RE) activity, such as liver and spleen, with only very limited accumulation in other major organs such as lung, kidney, brain and gut. The uptake of liposomes by RE cells is a major obstacle to investigators wishing to "target" liposomes to other sites. However, this natural distribution is very advantageous if specific delivery to macrophages is contemplated.

The distribution of intravenously administered liposomes is affected by their physical size, composition, charge, and the size of the inoculum. Although minor variations in distribution patterns can be achieved by altering these parameters, the majority of circulating

liposomes bind to and are endocytosed by cells of the RE system,
principally those located in the liver, spleen and lymph nodes.
Limited passage of small liposomes into organ parenchyma occurs in
organs that contain open sinusoidal capillaries (liver) but not in
organs that contain continuous capillaries (lungs). In addition,
circulating polymorphonuclear cells or monocytes are also capable of
engulfing liposomes. Thus, liposomes are selectively removed from
the circulation by active phagocytosis by free or fixed phagocytic
cells, and not by transcapillary passage. This natural fate of
liposomes can be used to target, albeit passively, immunomodulators
to cells of the RE system, and thereby result in their activation to
the tumoricidal state.

The role of macrophages in host defense against infections and
neoplasms has attracted increasing attention in the last several
years. There is a growing body of evidence that activated macrophages
are able to distinguish between tumorigenic and nontumorigenic cells,
and to kill tumor cells exhibiting various phenotypes, including
resistance to other host defense mechanisms and various anticancer
drugs. Macrophages can be activated to the tumoricidal state by a
diverse array of natural and synthetic materials, although most are
unsuitable as therapeutic modalities for macrophage activation in
vivo. For example, Mycobacteria, Corynebacteria, and Nocardia cell
walls interact directly with macrophages to induce activation.
However, the chemical constituents responsible for activation are
poorly understood, and their use in vivo is accompanied by significant toxicity with the notable exceptions of the synthetic moeity N-
acetyl-muramyl-L-alanyl-D-isoglutamine (MDP), which is the minimal
structural unit of Mycobacteria that has immune-potentiating
activity, and the recently introduced lipophilic MDP derivative N-
acetyl-muramyl-L-alanyl-D-isoglutanyl-L-alanyl-phosphatidylethanol-
amine (MTP-PE). Although MDP influences several macrophage functions
in vitro, comparable effects have not been observed in vivo because
it is cleared extremely rapidly after parenteral administration.
Even when injected in very high doses, MDP fails to induce significant macrophage-mediated antitumor activity because it is rapidly
cleared from the circulation. Consequently, efficient therapeutic

activation of macrophages in vivo requires that the agent be capable
of activating macrophages, irrespective of the "normal" physiological
pathways of the drug. Indeed, studies carried out in our laboratory
over the past several years suggest that liposomes can be used as
carrier vehicles for macrophage-activating agents in situ.

We have given particular attention to the feasibility of using
liposome-encapsulated immunomodulators (lymphokines, MDP, gamma
interferons, etc. etc.) to mobilize and activate tumoricidal macrophages in the lung, since this organ is a major site for metastatic
disease. To increase incorporation of liposomes into pulmonary macrophages, we have screened a wide range of liposomes of differing size,
surface charge and lipid composition for their ability to localize in
the lung after i.v. injection of mice. Large (0.5-10 μ diameter)
MLV, large unilamellar vesicles (LUV) and large reverse evaporation
vesicles (REV) liposomes arrest in the lung more efficiently than
small (300-800 Å) SUV liposomes of identical composition. Charged
liposomes are retained in the lung more efficiently than neutral
phosphatidylcholine (PC) liposomes. Optimal localization and retention in the lung without toxicity was obtained with negatively-
charged liposomes prepared from phosphatidylserine (PS) and PC (3:7
mole ratio). Negatively-charged LUV prepared from PS alone were
efficient in localizing in the lung, but their usefulness was limited
by systemic and pulmonary toxicity.

Toxicity studies in which MLV liposomes (PS/PC) containing
encapsulated lymphokines or MDP were injected i.v. into mice or
beagle dogs have failed to reveal any adverse reactions in recipient
animals even after large numbers of repeated injections.

IN VIVO ACTIVATION OF TUMORICIDAL PROPERTIES IN MACROPHAGES BY
LIPOSOME-ENCAPSULATED IMMUNOMODULATORS

Since negatively-charged MLV prepared from PS and PC (3:7 mole
ratio) localize in the lung parenchyma more efficiently than neutral
MLV liposomes consisting of PC alone, we have examined the relative
ability of these two liposomes to activate macrophages in situ. Both
PS/PC and PC MLV liposomes containing lymphokines (but not normal
lymphocyte supernatants or saline) can render alveolar macrophages

(AM) tumoricidal following in vitro incubation. Such was not the case for in vivo activation. AM harvested from mice 4 or 24 hr after i.v. injection of liposomes exhibited a higher level of cytotoxicity (as measured by an in vitro assay) if the macrophages were obtained from mice injected with PS/PC MLV. AM obtained from mice injected with PC MLV-encapsulated lymphokines or MDP were not tumoricidal. The failure of PC-encapsulated lymphokines or MDP to render AM tumoricidal in vivo following i.v. liposome injection to a level comparable to PS/PC encapsulated immunomodulators must be related to the increased efficiency of the latter liposomes to be arrested and retained in the lung microcirculation.

IN VIVO AUGMENTATION OF PULMONARY AND HEPATIC NK CELL ACTIVITY BY LIPOSOME-ENCAPSULATED MTP-PE

In addition to the activation of macrophages, the intravenous injection of liposomes containing MTP-PE also augments intrastitial NK cell activity in lung and liver, but not in the spleen or peripheral blood. Moreover, MLV containing MTP-PE did not augment splenic NK cells activity in vitro. These findings suggest that the augmentation of liver and lung NK cell activity was not due to the direct effect of the MLV-MTP-PE, but rather to a possible monokine liberated by liposome activated macrophages. Augmentation of pulmonary NK cell activity could be demonstrated by nonspecific immunoprophylaxis studies of experimental metastasis. Liposome generated augmentation of pulmonary NK cell activity could be reduced by pretreatment of mice with anti-asialo GM_1 antibodies. Collectively then, it appears that the augmentation of organ associated NK cell activity by liposomes containing MTP-PE could be important in the prophylaxis of hematogenous metastasis.

The ability to activate cells of the macrophage-histiocyte series in situ with lymphokine- or MDP-encapsulated liposomes is attractive for several reasons. Liposomes are nonimmunogenic, and the formation of granulomas and elicitation of allergic reactions commonly associated with the systemic administration of other immune adjuvants can be avoided. Moreover, neoplasms are known to be heterogeneous, and contain subpopulations of cells with different biological characteristics. Since, at least in vitro, tumoricidal macrophages can destroy tumor cells independently of other phenotypic characteristics, the in vivo activation of macrophages to develop tumoricidal properties might be useful toward inhibition or destruction of cancer metastases.

Spontaneous lymph node and pulmonary metastases were produced in mice by implanting B16-BL6 melanoma cells into their posterior foot-pads. Four to five weeks later, when the tumors reached 10-15 mm in diameter, the mice were anesthetized, and the tumor-bearing leg, including the popliteal lymph node, was amputated at the midfemur. Intravenous treatment with liposomes (2.5 μmol lipid/dose) begain 3 days later, and was repeated twice weekly for 4 weeks (8 injections). Seventy percent of mice treated with liposomes containing immunomodulators (MDP, lymphokines or both) survived at least 200 days, whereas only 5% of control mice survived. Thus, it appears that treatment of tumor-bearing mice with liposomes containing immunomodulators results in more effective systemic activation of macrophages and leads to the eradication of spontaneous pulmonary metastases.

Involvement of Macrophages in Disease States.

The mononuclear phagocyte system serves a primary function in host defense against a variety of microorganisms. Because of its scavenger activity, the macrophage plays an important role in resistance to diseases as diverse as, but not limited to, leishmaniasis, trypanosomiasis, malaria, tuberculosis, syphilis, brucellosis, salmonellosis, listeriosis, toxoplasmosis, histiocytosis, cryptococcosis, schistosomiasis, and leprosy. In many instances, however, facultative intracellular parasites are not destroyed by macrophages, but are able to survive and proliferate within their cytoplasm. This chronic presence of the parasite further stimulates macrophage influx to the infected site, resulting frequently in severe granulomatous lesions. An obvious example of this category in man is tuberculosis, in which there may be extensive multiplication of Mycobacteria within macrophages before cellular immunity develops. Neoplastic disorders of histiocytes include monocytic leukemia and histiocytosis X. Lysosomal storage diseases result when macrophages are unable to deal with phagocytosed organic material due to a deficiency of the appropriate enzyme. Thus, in Gaucher's disease, a lack of glucocerebrosidase leads to the accumulation of glucocerebroside in hepatic and splenic histiocytes. This wide variety of diseases may be treated by systemic administration of an appropriate drug or drugs encapsulated within liposomes during the intramacrophage phase of pathogenesis.

The targeting of liposome-encapsulated agents to phagocytic cells may offer a way to overcome the toxicity of drugs effective againt macrophage-associated diseases. Many of these drugs have toxic side effects that limit their use, and direct targeting of an agent to the site of action can allow significant reductions in the required drug concentrations, while concomitantly producing therapeutic drug concentrations in the infected cell. Indeed, high local levels of these drugs in cells of the macrophage series probably can be achieved by intravenous administration of liposomes containing or composed of these agents.

SELECTED REFERENCES

Interferon
 Friedman, R.M. and Vogel, S.N. Interferons with special emphasis on
 the immune system. Adv Immunol. 34:97-133, 1983.
 Maluish, A.E., Leavitt, R., Sherwin, S.A., Oldham, R.K. and Herberman,
 R.B. Effects of recombinant interferon-α on immune function in
 cancer patients. JBRM. 2:470-481, 1983.
 Smalley, R.V. and Oldham, R.K. Interferon as a biological response
 modifying agent in clinical trials. JBRM. 2:401-408, 1983.
 Toy, J.L. The interferons. Clin. Exp. Immunol. 54:1-13, 1983.
 Priestman, T.J. Interferon: an anti-cancer agent? Cancer Treat.
 Rev. 6:223-237, 1979.
 Brunda, M.J. and Rosenbaum, D. Modulation of murine natural killer
 cell activity in vitro and in vivo by recombinant human interferons.
 Cancer Res. 44:597-601, 1984.

MVE-2
 Carrano, R.A., Kinoshita, F.K., Imondi, A.R. and Iuliucci, J.D. MVE-
 2: preclinical pharmacology and toxicology. In: E.M. Hersh (eds.),
 Augmenting Agents in Cancer Therapy, pp. 345. New York: Raven
 Press, 1981.
 Milas, L., Hersh, E.M. and Hunter, N. Therapy of artificial and
 spontaneous metastases of murine tumors with maleic anhydride-divinyl
 ether-2. Cancer Res. 41:2378-2385, 1981.
 Chirigos, M.A. and Stylos, W.A. Immunomodulatory effect of various
 molecular-weight maleic anhydride-divinyl ethers and other agents
 in vivo. Cancer Res. 40:1967-1972, 1980.
 Talmadge, J.E., Maluish, A.E., Collins, M., Schneider, M., Herberman,
 R.B., Oldham, R.K. and Wiltrout, R.H. Immunomodulation and antitumor
 effects of MVE-2 in mice. JBRM. 3:000-000, 1984.
 Wiltrout, R.H., Mathieson, B.J., Talmadge, J.E., Reynolds, C.W., Zhang,
 S-R., Herberman, R.B. and Ortaldo, J.R. Augmentation of organ-
 associated natural killer activity by biological response modifiers.
 J. Exp. Med. 160:1431-1449, 1984.

Poly ICLC
 Talmadge, J.E., Adams, J., Phillips, H., Collins, M., Lenz, B.,
 Schneider, M. and Chirigos, M. Immunotherapeutic potential of
 polyinosinic - polycytidylic acid - poly L lysine, carboxymethyl
 cellulose in tumor models. Cancer Res. (In Press)
 Talmadge, J.E., Adams, J., Phillips, H., Collins, M., Lenz, B.,
 Schneider, M., Schlick, E., Ruffmann, R., Wiltrout, R.H. and Chirigos,
 M.A. Immunomodulatory effects of polyinosinic - polycytidylic acid -
 poly L lysine, carboxymethyl cellulose in mice. Cancer Res. (In Press)
 Chirigos, M.A., Papademetriou, V., Bartocci, A., Read, E. and Levy,
 H.B. Immune response modifying activity in mice of polyinosinic:
 polycytidylic acid stabilized with poly-L-lysine, in carboxymethylcellulose (poly-ICLC). Int. J. Immunopharmac. 3:329-337, 1981.
 Levine, A.S., Sivulich, M., Wiernik, P.H. and Levy, H.B. Initial
 clinical trials in cancer patients of polyriboinosinic-polyribocytidylic acid stabilized with poly-L-lysine, in carboxymethylcellulose
 [poly(ICLC)], a highly effective interferon inducer. Cancer Res.
 39:1645-1650, 1979.

Djeu, J.Y., Heinbaugh, J.A., Vieira, W.D., Holden, H.T and Herberman, R.B. The effect of immunopharmacological agents on mouse natural cell-mediated cytotoxicity and on its augmentation by poly I:C. Immunopharmacology 1:231-244, 1979.

Levy, H.B. and Riley, F.L. A comparison of immune modulating effects of interferon and interferon inducers. Academic Press 8:303-321, 1

Thymosin

Zatz, M.M., Low, T.L.K. and Goldstein, A.L. Role of thymosin and other thymic hormones in T-cell differentiation. Biological Respon in Cancer. 1:219, 1982.

Marshall, G.D., Thurman, G.B. and Goldstein, A.L. Regulation of in vitro generation of cell-mediated cytotoxicity. II. Characterizatio of thymosin-induced suppressor T cells. Immunopharmacology 2:301-3 1980.

Talmadge, J.E., Uithoven, K.A., Lenz, B.F. and Chirigos, M. Immunomodulation and therapeutic characterization of thymosin fract five. Cancer Immunol Immunother. 00:000-000, 1984

Low, T.L.K., Thurman, G.B., Chincarini, C., McClure, J.E., Marshall, G.D., Hu, S.K. and Goldstein, A.L. Current status of thymosin research: Evidence for the existence of a family of thymic factors that control T-cell maturation. Ann NY Acd Sci 33:48.

Schulof, R.S. and Goldstein, A.L. Clinical applications of thymosin and other thymic hormones: Recent Advances in Clinical Immunology. Thompson and Rose. (eds) Churchill Livingstone NY, 1983.

Interleukin 2

Talmadge, J.E. Immunoregulation and immunostimulation of murine lymphocytes by recombinant human interleukin 2. JBRM. (In Press).

Farrar, J.J., Benjamin, W.R., Hilfiker, M.L., Howard, M., Farrar, W.L. and Fuller-Farrar, J. The biochemistry, biology, and role of interleukin 2 in the induction of cytotoxic T cell and antibody-forming B cell responses. Immunological Rev. 63, 1982.

Smith, K.A., Baker, P.E., Gillis, S. and Ruscetti, F.W. Functional and molecular characteristics of T-cell growth factor. Molecular Immunology 17:579-589, 1979.

Cheever, M.A., Greenberg, P.D., Fefer, A. and Gillis, S. Augmentatio of the anti-tumor therapeutic efficacy of long-term cultured T lymphocytes by in vivo adminstration of purified interleukin 2. J. Exp. Med. 155:968-980, 1982.

McGrogan, M., Doyle, M., Kawasaki, E., Koths, K. and Mark, D.F. Biological activity of recombinant human interleukin-2 produced in Escherichia coli. Science 223:1412, 1984.

OK-432

Murayama, T., Natsuume-Sakai, S., Ryoyama, K. and Koshimura, S. Studies of the properties of a streptococcal preparation, OK-432 (NSC-B116209), as an immunopotentiator. Cancer Immunol Immunother. 12:141-146, 1982.

Wakasugi, H., Kasahara, T., Minato, N., Hamuro, J., Miyata, M. and Morioka, Y. In vitro potentiation of human natural killer cell activity by a streptococcal preparation, OK-432: interferon and interleukin-2 participation in the stimulation with OK-432. JNCI. 69:807, 1982.

Uchida, A. and Micksche, M. Intrapleural administration of OK-432 in cancer patients: Activation of NK cells and reduction of suppressor cells. Int. J. Cancer. 31:1-5, 1983.

Micksche, M., Kokron, O. and Uchida, A. Clinical and immunopharmacological studies with OK-432, a streptococcal preparation. Elsevier Biomedical Press B.V. Current Concepts in Human Immunology and Cancer Immunomodulation. B. Serrou et al. 1982.

Endotoxin
    Morrison, D.C. and Ryan, J.L. Bacterial endotoxins and host immune responses. Adv. Immunol. 28:294-374, 1979.
    Ribi, E.E., Granger, D.L., Milner, K.C. and Strain, S.M. Brief communication: Tumor regression caused by endotoxins and mycrobacterial fractions. J. Natl. Cancer Inst. 55:1253, 1975.
    Ribi, E. Beneficial modification of the endotoxin molecule. JBRM. 3:1-9, 1984.

Lentinan
    Rose, W.C., Reed, F.C., Siminoff, P. and Bradner, W.T. Immunotherapy of Madison 109 lung carcinoma and other murine tumors using lentinan. Cancer Res. 44:1368-1373, 1984.
    Fruehauf, J.P., Bonnard, G.D. and Herberman, R.B. The effect of lentinan on production of interleukin-1 by human monocytes. Immunopharmacol. 5:65-74, 1982.
    Chihara, G and Taguchi, T. Lentinan: Biological activities and possible clinical use. J. Immunol. & Immunopharmacol. 2:93-104, 1982.
    Chihara, G., Maeda, Y.Y. and Hamuro, J. Current status and perspectives of immunomodulators of microbial origin. Int. J. Tiss. Reac. 3:207-225, 1982.

Muramyl Dipeptide
    Chedid, L. and Morin, A. Current status of muramyl peptides. Elsevier Biomedical Press B.V. Current Concepts in Human Immunology and Cancer Immunomodulation B. Serrou et al. p.535, 1982.
    Matter, A. The effects of muramyldipeptide (MDP) in cell-mediated immunity. Cancer Immunol. Immunother. 6:201-210, 1979.
    Adam, A. and Lederer, E. Muramyl peptides: Immunomodulators, sleep factors, and vitamin. Med Res Rev. 4:111-152, 1984.

FK-565
    Mine, Y., Yokota, Y., Wakai, Y., Fukuda, S., Nishida, M., Goto, S. and Kuwahara, S. Immunoactive peptides, FK-156 and FK-565:I. Enhancement of host resistance to microbial infection in mice. J Antibiotics. 36: 1045-1051, 1983.
    Izumi, S., Nakahara, K., Gotoh, T., Hashimoto, S., Kino, T., Okuhara, M., Aoki, H. and Imanaka, H. Antitumor effects of novel immunoactive peptides, FK-156 and its synthetic derivative. J Antibiotics. 36:156-174, 1983.
    Kino, T., Hashimoto, S., Nakahara, K., Gotoh, T., Aoki, H. and Imanaka, H. Inhibition of tumor metastasis by selective of natural killer cells by immunoactive peptides, FK-565 and FK-091. JBRM (In Press)

Azimexone
Bicker, U. Immunomodulating effects of BM 12.531 in animals and tolerance in man. Cancer Treatment Reports. 62:1987, 1978.
Bruley-Rosset, M., Hercend, T., Martinez, J., Rappaport, H. and Mathe, G. Prevention of spontaneous tumors of aged mice by immunopharmacologic manipulation: Study of immune antitumor mechanisms. JNCI. 66:1113, 1981.
Stylos, W.A., Chirigos, M.A., Papademetriou, V. and Lauer, L. The immunomodulatory effect of BM 12.531 (azimexon) on normal or tumored mice: in vitro and in vivo studies. J Immunopharmcol. 2:113-132, 1

Bestatin
Blomgren, H., Edsmyr, F., Esposti, P-L., Naslund, I. and Strender, L-E. Influence of bestatin, a new immunomodifier, on human lymphoid cells. Elsevier Biomedical Press B.V. Current Concepts in Human Immunology and Cancer Immunomodulation B. Serrou et al. 593 1982.
Schorlemmer, H.U., Bosslet, K. and Sedlacek. H.H. Ability of the immunomodulating dipeptide bestatin to activate cytotoxic mononucle phagocytes. Cancer Res. 43:4148-4153, 1983.
Umezawa, H. Small molecular microbial products enhancing immune response. Antibiot. Chemother. 24:9-18, 1978.

Alkyl lysophospholipids
Berdel, W.E., Bausert, W.R.E., Fink, U., Rastetter, J. and Munder, P.G. Anti-tumor action of alkyl-lysophospholipids. Anticancer Res 1:345-352, 1981.
Berdel, W.E. Antineoplastic activity of synthetic lysophospholipid analogs. Blut. 44:71-78, 1982.
Munder, P.G., Modolell, M., Bausert, W., Oettgen, H.F. and Westphal, O. Alkyllysophospholipids in cancer therapy. Raven Press, New York, 441, 1981.

Liposomes
Poste, G., Bucana, C., Raz, A., Bugelski, P., Kirsh, R. and Fidler, I.J. Analysis of the fate of systemically administered liposomes and implications for their use in drug delivery. Cancer Res. 42: 1412-1422, 1982.
Fidler, I.J. The in situ induction of tumoricidal activity in alveolar macrophages by liposomes containing muramyl dipeptide is a thymus-independent process. J Immunol. 127:1719, 1981.
Fidler, I.J., Sone, S., Fogler, W.E. and Barnes, Z.L. Eradication of spontaneous metastases and activation of alveolar macrophages by intravenous injection of liposomes containing muramyl dipeptide. Proc Natl Acad Sci. 78:1680-1684, 1981.
Sone, S., Mutsuura, S., Ogawara, M. and Tsubura, E. Potentiating effect of muramyl dipeptide and its lipophylic analog encapsulated in liposomes on tumor cell killing by human monocytes. J Immunol. 132: 2105, 1984.

CLINICAL CORRELATIONS

INTRODUCTION

A variety of clinical trials have now been performed with certain of the compounds that have been tested in the Preclinical Screening Laboratory. Although the number and extent of these clinical trials are still limited, a data base is emerging on clinical activity for a few of the compounds evaluated in the screening program. The purpose of this chapter will be to look at those compounds where correlations can be drawn and to attempt to determine whether the activities seen in the screening program are reflected in the clinical trials. This is not a straight forward task since few phase II or phase III clinical trials have been undertaken to provide data on therapeutic efficiency. In addition, immunomonitoring during phase I trials is not universal and no uniform assays or approach are recognized. Thus, of necessity clinical - preclinical correlations are limited and, at present of a somewhat superfical nature. The BRMP is developing a unified approach to immunomonitoring during clinical trials and we hope that similar approaches will be established for most clinical trials. The Preclinical Screening Laboratory and Biological Response Modifiers Program are undertaking a comprehensive literature review with a detailed analysis and evaluation of the immunomodulatory and therapeutic properties of BRMs. Obviously, there are two major correlations to be considered. The first is to look for evidence of in vivo inhibition of tumor growth in the preclinical models and correlate that with antitumor activity in man. The second correlation involves the biological response modifying activity of these compounds, where one can attempt to correlate observations on modulation of biological responses in the preclinical screen with changes in the biological responses observed in clinical studies. Unfortunately, it is not clear that biological response modification, as reflected in our assays, correlates directly with antitumor response.

179

Table 1

Antitumor Activity
of the Alpha Interferons

Tumors	Average Response Rates
Lymphoma	
"Good Prognosis" lymphoma	40-60%
"Poor Prognosis" lymphoma	0-20%
Myeloma	10-25%
Chronic Leukemias	
Lymphocytic	0-25%
Myelocytic	50-70%
Hairy Cell	80%
Melanoma	5-20%
Breast Cancer	0-40%
Renal Cancer	10-40%
Kaposi's Sarcoma	20-40%
Ovarian Cancer	10-20%

In fact, with the clinical studies of IFN there is some evidence that
the antitumor response and the immunomodulating response may be observed
at very different dose levels (1,2). This being the case, it is important to be cautious while making these correlations. It may well be
that an excellent correlation in biological response modification between the preclinical model and man might be seen without any concomitant
evidence of clinical antitumor activity. Such correlations would be
of lesser importance than those in which preclinical activity might be
reflected in a clear antitumor response in the clinical trials. However,
few clinical trials are predicated on protocols to obtain an optimal
immunomodulatory dose (OID) rather than a maximum tolerated dose (MTD).
We suggest that future clinical trials should be designed to specifically
address such questions. Thus, this chapter will focus on clinical
observations and will attempt to correlate these observations with the
data base accumulating from the Preclinical Screen.

INTERFERONS

    Two recent review articles have very completely summarized most of
the clinical trials using alpha, beta, and gamma interferon (3,4).
These reviews were based on information available up until 1984 and are
current with respect to the interferon clinical trial data base.
Obviously, ongoing phase II and III trials with alpha interferon and
phase I and II trials with gamma and beta interferons will continue to
enlarge the data base during the coming years. However, it is clear
that significant antitumor activity of the alpha interferons has been
seen in a variety of cancers (Table 1). In contrast to the responses
seen and summarized in Table 1, little antitumor activity has been seen
for more common malignancies such as those of the colon or lung (3-6).

    Two questions emerge. What is the correlation of the antitumor ac-
tivity observed in clinical trials with the immunomodulatory responses
being measured? What is the correlation between the antitumor responses
seen in man and the preclinical antitumor activity observed in the screening program? There is no direct answer to the first question. In some.
but not all, of the phase I-II trials of certain lymphomas, more interferon appears to be better in inducing antitumor responses (7,8). However, for NK cell augmentation the most effective biological response

modifying dose appears to be much lower (1,9-11) than the MTD. In virtually none of the clinical trials performed to date have the doses producing the maximum biological response been defined, much less correlations undertaken, with the doses producing the maximum antitumor response. Interferons also have direct antiproliferative activity which also provides a likely mechanism of action underlying the clinical antitumor activity. With respect to the second question, the analysis is complex. Recombinant interferons of the type used in the clinic have had minimal activity on rodent cells, making any direct correlation impossible. In fact, most of the interferons used in human clinical studies have little or no activity on rodent cells and would not be expected to have significant antitumor activity in the preclinical screen in vitro or in animal tumor models. As is reviewed elsewhere in this monograph, cloned human interferons had little or no activity in the preclinical screen. The recombinant hybrid human interferon and mouse interferons that did have activity augmented macrophage cytotoxicity and NK activity as expected. In appropriate doses (50,000 U/animal) and schedules (biw) these agents had some activity against spontaneous and experimental metastases.

The data on beta and gamma interferons are complicated by some of the same considerations discussed above for the alpha interferons. Insufficient clinical data are available to make any correlations with the preclinical screen activity for these compounds. In fact, only gamma interferon has been entered into the screening program and it has not yet been fully tested for antitumor activity. It will be of interest to make the correlations with this form of interferon since it appears to have greater macrophage activating properties and perhaps antiproliferative, capacity on a unit-per-unit basis when compared with the alpha interferons.

INTERFERON INDUCERS

The most effective nonviral inducers of interferon have been the double-stranded ribonucleic acids. Of these, polyriboinosinic: polyribocytidylic acid (poly I:C), an effective inducer in rodent systems, is a very poor interferon inducer because of rapid hydrolysis in human serum.

In order to circumvent this problem, a hydrophilic complex formed
between poly-L-lysine and carboxymethylcellulose was combined with
poly I:C to produce poly ICLC, which is soluble in saline and partially
resistant to hydrolysis in human sera (12). A number of phase I trials
using poly ICLC administered by 30- to 60-minute infusions have been
performed to evaluate several schedules. Toxicity has been significant,
but occasional antitumor responses (in acute leukemia, multiple myeloma,
renal cell carcinoma, and chronic lymphatic leukemia) have been seen
(13). Augmentation of both NK activity and macrophage activation have
been associated with interferon induction in humans. However, at dose
levels that are tolerable, high levels of serum interferon activity are
not induced (14). Several other small molecular weight compounds may
also induce interferon production (15). Interest in these compounds
has waned with the development and ready availability through genetic
engineering of a number of interferon molecules.

Preclinical screen data indicate that poly ICLC can stimulate NK and
macrophage activity and that this compound does have in vivo activity in
rodent tumor model systems. A comparison of antitumor activity and immunomodulation between the screen and man can be made for this compound, although it is difficult to link either activity to interferon levels. Poly
ICLC has not been sufficiently tested in phase II trials to allow the comparison of clinical and preclinical antitumor activity. In the screen,
there is a clear dissociation between an OID and the MTD for this compound.
Indeed, in both the preclinical screen and in the clinic therapeutic
activity has not been observed at the MTD.

MVE-2 (maleic vinyl ether), a pyran copolymer, has received fairly
extensive preclinical evaluation both as an immunomodulator and as an
antitumor agent in animal models. Preclinical studies indicated that
this agent activates macrophages and induces interferon production. When
administered under the appropriate experimental conditions, including
attention to the site of administration and timing in relation to the
tumor cell transplant, definite antitumor activity can be demonstrated
in peritoneal tumor model systems (16,17). However, systemic administration directed against preexistent metastatic disease has not demonstrated therapeutic activity. Recently completed phase I trials in
humans with advanced cancer have indicated that this agent has little

consistent immunostimulatory capability in patients with large tumor burdens. No substantial antitumor effects were seen in these phase I trials (17,18).

T CELL IMMUNOREGULATORS
Thymosins.

The thymosins are polypeptides produced by the epithelial cells of the thymus gland. They have been extracted from calf thymus gland (20) and partially purified for clinical use. Thymic extracts will immunologically reconstitute neonatally thymectomized mice (21). Recent evaluations have pointed to a general developmental role for the thymosins in the maturation of T cells (22).

Clinical studies with thymosin fraction 5 during the late 1970s demonstrated an immunorestorative function in selected immunodeficient children. This clinical benefit was correlated with an in vitro augmentation of the mixed lymphocyte reaction (MLR) (23). Subsequent randomized trails in adults with small cell carcinoma of the lung and in head and neck squamous cell carcinoma demonstrated an improved survival for those patients receiving thymosin fraction 5 (24,25). This was associated with restored delayed hypersensitivity and an improvement in the MLR.

More recently, both thymosin fraction 5 and the synthetically produced thymosin alpha-1 have been evaluated in phase I and early phase II trials (26). Very little toxicity and some immunomodulatory activity has been ascribed to both of these products. Occasional objective responses were seen with thymosin fraction 5 in patients with renal cell carcinoma (27). In a small randomized placebo-controlled trial in patients receiving radiation therapy for primary stage I-III non-small cell carcinoma of the lung, two different schedules of thymosin alpha-1 induced an improved disease-free interval (28). This improvement was associated with an improvement in the MLR in some (28) but not all trials (29). Confirmatory trials in both of these diseases are underway.

In the screen, thymosin preparations do induce higher levels of T cell activity and differentiation. Significant in vivo activity against experimental and spontaneous metastasis was observed at doses in the high range of those needed to affect T cell activity. Thus, the correlation of in vitro biological response modification and in vivo activity appears straight forward in the rodent models. Like poly ICLC, thymosin's activity in the screen has been reflected in the clinic but it is premature to discuss therapeutic activity with these BRMs.

Interleukin 2 (IL-2).

IL-2, produced by helper T cells in the presence of T cell stimulants (lectins, allogeneic cells, and/or soluble antigen) will stimulate and maintain the growth of normal activated T cells (30) in vitro. A number of laboratories have demonstrated or have begun to identify the various subpopulations of T lymphocytes involved in the specific cytotoxic antitumor response and have begun to manipulate these populations with exogenously administered IL-2 (31,32). Specifically, cytotoxic antitumor T cells or LAK cells have been grown in long-term culture with IL-2 and such cells when introduced intravenously in small solid tumor models have induced cures. Such cells have also been given to patients in exploratory early phase clinical studies. The BRM effects and clinical activities of IL-2-induced cells are described in detail in a recent symposium (33). IL-2 has a very short serum half-life and it is as yet unclear whether it has any antitumor activity since early phase clinical trials have just begun (33). In the screen, IL-2 augmented certain T cell functions, NK cells, and macrophages. Its activity in the peritoneal compartments was more significant, suggesting the need to consider analogous trials in man. There are insufficient data available to attempt correlation between in vitro activation by IL-2 and antitumor activity.

NATURAL PRODUCTS, BACTERIAL EXTRACTS AND SYNTHETIC IMMUNOMODULATORS

Bacterial products

The era of nonspecific immunotherapy began with Mathé's report in the late 1960s of the clinical efficacy of BCG, in which both the duration of response and survival of children with acute lymphocytic leukemia were prolonged following repeated administration of BCG (34). The minimal active component in these extracts for adjuvant activity is muramyldipeptide (MDP) (35). Attempts are now under way to further define and synthesize analogues in order to produce pure and reproducibly effective pharmaceutical products (36,37). Clinical trials with BCG and other bacteria such as C. parvum have not yielded conclusive results (38,39), and the Preclinical Screen testing has been confined to MDP.

MDP has proven to be a powerful activator of macrophages, especially when encapsulated in liposomes. Unfortunately, no clinical data are available as yet due to the pyrogenic properties of MDP and thus these are no correlations of screen activity with clinical trials.

OK-432 (Picibanil) is a lyophilized preparation of a nonvirulent strain of Streptococcus and has been evaluated in a number of clinical trials in Japan. This preparation augments NK and T cell cytotoxicity and leads to macrophage activation in rodent models, activities which have been confirmed in the Preclinical Screen. Clinically, the material is locally therapeutically active in about 50% of patients with pleural or peritoneal effusions, demonstrating efficacy in those patients whose effusions contain tumor cells (40). When administered intravenously or intramuscularly, NK cytotoxicity is augmented, monocytes are activated, and clinical benefit (prolonged survival) has been reported in patients with lymphoma, gastric carcinoma, and non-small cell cancer (41). In the screen, OK-432 was active in experimental and spontaneous metastasis models, though less so than poly ICLC in reducing the median number of metastases and prolonging survival. Additionally, some activity was also seen in the autochthonous models. These positive results were at doses which induced heightened NK and macrophage activity. As with the T cell active agents discussed earlier, the number of clinical antitumor responses to systemically administered OK-432 are insufficient to allow definitive correlations. The local antitumor activity may be immune-based, but given the inflammatory properties of this compound, local activity may simply be due to adhesions from an inflammatory response much as is seen when tetracycline is administered into peritoneal effusions.

Following the initial demonstration several years ago of antitumor activity in fungal cell wall preparations, a great many active poly-saccharide components of fungal and bacterial origin have been identified Several of these have undergone clinical evaluation. While these poly-saccharides possess the advantage over whole organisms of being chemically defined and potentially synthesizable, they may have significantly less activity than the whole organism (42). Glucan from Saccharomyes cerevisiae, Krestin from a Basidiomycetes, and Lentinan, a beta glucan from aqueous extracts of mushrooms, are perhaps the most well known

agents in this class. These agents activate macrophages and stimulate
T cell function but are not potent inducers of interferon production
nor augmentors of NK cytotoxicity. They have been reported to have
antitumor activity in several murine models (43,44). These immunomodulatory and antitumor activities have been confirmed in the BRM screen.
However, the latter effects have been modest and always less striking
than the positive controls. Although many studies have been done in
the clinic by Japanese investigators, many of the reports involve the
use of these agents as adjuvants. Thus, it is difficult to establish
a clinical level of effectiveness to correlate with the laboratory
observations (45,46).

Chemical immunomodulators.

Several inhibitors of enzyme activity (aminopeptidase, phosphatase,
and esterase) normally associated with cell membranes have been associated
with immunomodulation. These small molecular weight compounds have been
extracted and purified from the culture filtrates of several Streptomyces
strains and evaluated both preclinically and clinically (47). Bestatin,
the compound that has been most extensively studied clinically, has been
characterized chemically, has shown immunomodulatory capabilities, and
has demonstrated antitumor effects in several murine systems. It has
undergone extensive clinical trials in Japan and has been evaluated in
a phase I study in Europe (48,49). Some augmentation of delayed hypersensitivity and of NK cytotoxicity has been reported in certain subsets
of patients. Further, in at least four randomized clinical trials in
patients with relatively low tumor burdens (squamous cell carcinoma of
the skin, malignant melanoma, superficial bladder tumors, and acute non-
lymphocytic leukemia), bestatin has been associated with improved survival (50-52). In the Preclinical Screen, Bestatin has demonstrated
adjuvant activity and macrophage stimulatory properties. Bestatin has
also demonstrated therapeutic activity directed against experimental
and spontaneous B16-BL6 metastases as well as NMU induced mammary tumors.
For other agents such as azimexon, FK-565, N-137, ALP, and LPS (the
screening results of which are reviewed earlier in this monograph)
insufficient clinical data are available to draw correlations (53).

Liposome-encapsulated immunomodulators.

The preclinical data on this approach have been reviewed (54-56).

While this approach appears very promising in preclinical models and
the screening data reviewed here are confirmatory, no clinical trials
have been done to validate the concept. Very early trials with liposomes
and liposomes containing antibiotics are underway but no activity data
have yet been reported.

SUMMARY AND CONCLUSIONS

Based on the observations available from the Preclinical Screen,
studies in other laboratories, and clinical trials, there is a strong par-
ellel between immunomodulatory activity in the Preclinical Screening Program and immunomodulatory activity in the clinic. As discussed earlier, a
insufficient data base is available to make any far-reaching conclusions,
but it is already clear that certain of these agents which have biological
activity in man also have biological activity in the screening program.
The difficulty arises in making precise correlations to the mechanisms
of action underlying the biological response modifying effects and the
observed antitumor effects. Interferons, if appropriately chosen for
species selectivity, are active in the screening program as biological
response modifiers and do demonstrate some antitumor effects. In the
clinic, induction of NK and macrophage activities is fairly consistent
and a number of antitumor responses have also been seen. Nonetheless,
interferons also have antiproliferative activities and the antitumor
effect may be secondary to the antiproliferative capability of this
compound rather than to its immunomodulatory role. However, further
studies are needed to clarify this issue.

The T cell active agents such as thymosin and interleukin 2 do
demonstrate the ability to induce changes in T cell maturation, and
they also show activity in the screening program. In addition, they
have evident activity as therapeutic agents in the preclincal models.
Unfortunately, the number of clinical responses seen with thymic
products has been too few to make any definite correlations. Interleukin 2 is only now entering clinical trials and it is too early for
such correlations to be considered. However, it is encouraging that
some clinical responses have been seen with thymic preparations and
further studies are warranted to define the activity and mechanisms of
action of these compounds. The doses used to induce antitumor effects

have been in the same range as for those that induce immunomodulatory effects.

Interferon inducers have shown a consistent ability to increase NK activity and stimulate macrophage cytotoxicity. In clinical studies the immunostimulatory effects and the clinical antitumor effects have been inconsistent. Because some antitumor responses have been seen with poly ICLC, it would be reasonable to design careful clinical studies attempting to correlate the biological response modifying effects of this compound with its antitumor activity.

With all of the other agents tested in the screen and evaluated in the clinic, there are insufficient data to make even preliminary conclusions. It is ironic that the largest number of patients studied with some of these compounds, in sometimes randomized trials, has been in Japan and Europe. Because these studies look for survival and small statistical changes in end points, it will probably never be possible to correlate antitumor effects with biological response modifying effects in these studies. By virtue of the design of adjuvant studies which look for a decreased recurrence rate and an increased survival in large populations of patients, it will be difficult to make these correlations since one does not know for certain which patients had the antitumor effects. The goal for future clinical trials should be to measure biological response modifying effects on a patient-by patient basis and undertake comparisons with the biological response modifying effects and the antitumor effects for each individual patient.

The design of clinical trials for immunotherapy is a controversial subject (46). For those agents capable of inducing antitumor responses with clinically apparent disease, there is the real possibility of drawing correlations between antitumor responses and biological response modifying effects. However, for those agents that work only in the adjuvant setting, such comparisons will always be difficult. It is encouraging to note that certain forms of biotherapy can give antitumor responses in patients with clinically apparent disease, and it is for these agents and in these categories of patients that studies of mechanism of action can best be performed (2). As for chemotherapy, one could then design trials in patients with minimal disease using the principles garnered from patients with apparent disease. The criticism will always be that we may miss those agents which are active in minimal disease and inactive in clinically apparent disease. While this is a just criticism, it does not negate the approach of those who wish to explore agents with known antitumor activity (38). Ongoing trials with biologicals and biological response modifiers should further define their activity in the clinic. It is anticipated that these data will be helpful in making judgments regarding the usefulness of the NCI BRM Preclinical Screen. There are too few correlations possible to make such a judgment possible in 1984, but perhaps as soon as 1988 a very stringent review of these screening activities will be possible, giving those involved the opportunity to alter the screening program in a rational, scientifically based manner.

REFERENCES

1. Oldham, R.K. and Smalley, R.V. The role of interferon in the treatment of cancer. In: Interferon: Research, Clinical Application, and Regulatory Consideration (Eds. K.C. Zoon, P.C. Nogushi and T.Y. Liu), Elsevier Science Publishers, Amsterdam, 1984, pp. 191-205.
2. Oldham, R.K. Biologicals and biological response modifiers: Fourth modality of cancer treatment. Cancer Treat. Rep. 68:221-232, 1984.
3. Kirkwood, J.M. and Ernstoff, M.S. Interferons in the treatment of human cancer. J. Clin. Oncol. 12:336-352, 1984.
4. Bonnem, E.M. and Spiegel, R.J. Alpha interferon: Current status and future promise. J. Biol. Resp. Modif. 3(6), in press.
5. Sarna, G., Figlin, R. and Callaghan, M. Alpha (human leukocyte)-interferon as treatment for non-small cell carcinoma of the lung: A phase II trial. J. Biol. Resp. Modif. 2:343-347, 1983.
6. Neefe, J.R., Silgals, R., Ayoob, M. and Schein, P.S. Minimal activity of recombinant clone A interferon in metastatic colon cancer. J. Biol. Resp. Modif. 3:366-370, 1984.
7. Foon, K.A., Sherwin, S.A., Abrams, P.G., Longo, D.L., Fer, M.F., Stevenson, H.C., Ochs, J.J., Bottino, G.C., Schoenberger, C.S., Zeffren, J., Jaffe, E.S. and Oldham, R.K. Treatment of advanced non-Hodgkin's lymphoma with recombinant leukocyte A interferon. New Engl. J. Med. 11:1148-1152, 1984.
8. Bunn, P.A., Foon, K.A., Ihde, D.C., Longo, D.L., Eddy, J., Winkler, C.F., Veach, S.R., Zeffren, J., Sherwin, S. and Oldham, R.K. Recombinant leukocyte A interferon: An active agent in advanced cutaneous T-cell lymphomas. Ann. Intern. Med. 101:484-487, 1984.
9. Ozer, H., Gavigan, M., O'Malley, J., Thompson, D., Dadey, B., Nussbaum-Blumenson, A., Snider, C., Rudnick, S., Ferraresi, R., Norred, S. and Han, T. Immunomodulation by recombinant interferon-alpha 2 in a phase I trial in patients with lymphoproliferative malignancies. J. Biol. Resp. Modif. 2:499-515, 1983.

10. Herberman, R.B. and Thurman, G.B. Approaches to the immunological monitoring of cancer patients treated with natural or recombinant interferons. J. Biol. Resp. Modif. 2:548-562, 1983.

11. Smalley, R.V. and Oldham, R.K. Interferon as a biological response modifying agent in clinical trials. J. Biol. Resp. Modif. 2:401-408, 1984.

12. Levy, H.B., Baer, G., Baron, S., et al. A modified polyriboinosinic-polyribocytidylic acid complex that induces interferon in primates. J. Infect. Dis. 132:434-439, 1975.

13. Stringfellow, D.A. and Smalley, R.V. Interferon inducers for clinical use. In: In Vivo Application of Interferons (Eds. N. Finter and R. Oldham), Elsevier Science Publishers, Amsterdam, 1984, in press.

14. Levy, H.G., Stephen, E.S., Harrington, D., et al. Polynucleotides in the treatment of disease. In: Augmenting Agents in Cancer Therapy (Eds. E.M. Hersh, M.A. Chirigos and M. Mastrangelo), Raven Press, New York, 1981, pp. 135-150.

15. Stringfellow, D.A. Induction of interferon with low molecular weight compounds: fluorenone ester, ethers (tilorone), and pyrimidinones. Methods Enzymol. 78:262-284, 1981.

16. Chirigos, M.A. and Stylos WA. Immunomodulatory effect of various molecular-weight maleic anhydride-divinyl ethers and other agents in vivo. Cancer Res. 40:1967-1972, 1980.

17. Talmadge, J.R., Maluish, A.E., Collins, M., Schneider, M., Herberman, R.B., Oldham, R.K. and Wiltrout, R.H. Immunomodulation and antitumor effects of MVE-2 in mice. J. Biol. Resp. Modif. 2(6), in press.

18. Rios, A., Rosenblum, M., Powell, M. and Hersh, E. Phase I study of MVE-2 therapy in human cancer. Cancer Treat. Rep. 67:239-243, 1983.

19. Rinehart, J.J., Young, D.C. and Neidhart, J.A. Evaluation of the immunological and toxicological properties of MVE-2 in phase I trials. Cancer Res. 43:2358-2362, 1983.

20. Low, T., Thurman, G., McAdoo, M., et al. The chemistry and biology of thymosin. I. Isolation, characterization, and biological activities of thymosin alpha-1 and polypeptide beta-1 from calf thymus. J. Biol. Chem. 245:981-986, 1979.

21. Goldstein, A.L., Low, T.L.K., Thurman, G.B., et al. Current status of thymosin and other hormones of the thymus gland. Recent Progress in Hormone Research 37:369-415, 1981.

22. Thurman, G.B., Marshall, G.D., Low, T.L.K. and Goldstein, A. Structural studies and immunoregulatory role in host immunity. In: Thymus, Thymic Hormones and T Lymphocytes (Eds.) F. Aiuti and H. Wigzell), Academic Press, New York, 1980, pp. 175-185.

23. Wara, D., Barrett, D., Ammann, A. and Cowan, M. In vitro and in vivo enhancement of mixed lymphocyte culture reactivity by thymosin in patients with primary immunodeficiency disease. J. Pediatr. 97:66-71, 1980.

24. Cohen, M., Chretien, P., Ihde, D., et al. Thymosin fraction V and intensive combination chemotherapy. JAMA 241:1813-1815, 1979.

25. Wara, W., Neely, M., Ammann, A. and Wara, D. Biologic modification of immunologic parameters in head and neck cancer patients with thymosin fraction 5. In: Lymphokines and Thymic Hormones: Their Potential Utilization in Cancer Therapeutics (Eds. A. Goldstein and M.A. Chirigos), Raven Press, New York, 1981, pp. 257-262.

26. Dillman, R.O., Beauregard, J.C., Mendelsohn, J., Green, M.R., Howell, S. and Royston, I. Phase I trials of thymosin fraction 5 and thymosin alpha-1. J. Biol. Resp. Modif. 1:35-41, 1982.

27. Schulof, R.S., Lloyd, M.J., Ueno, W.M., Green, L.D. and Stallings, J.J. Phase II trial of thymosin fraction 5 in advanced renal cancer. J. Biol. Resp. Modif. 3:151-159, 1984.

28. Schulof, R.S., Lloyd, M., Cox, J. and Goldstein, A.L. Synthetic thymosin alpha-1 following mediastinal irradiation: A randomized trial in patients with locally advanced non-small cell lung cancer. Proc. ASCO 2:185, 1983.

29. Dillman, R.O., Beauregard, J.C., Zavanelli, M.I., Halliburton, B.L., Wormsley, S. and Royston, I. In vivo immune restoration in advanced cancer patients after administration of thymosin fraction 5 or thymosin alpha-1. J. Biol. Resp. Modif. 2:139-149, 1983.

30. Ruscetti, F.W. and Gallo, R.C. Human T-lymphocyte growth factor: Regulation of growth and function of T-lymphocytes. Blood 57:379-394, 1981.

31. Cheever, M.A., Greenberg, P.D., Fefer, A. and Gillis, S. Augmentatio of the anti-tumor therapeutic efficacy of long-term cultured T lymphc cytes by in vivo administration of purified interleukin-2. J. Exp. Med. 155:968-980, 1982.

32. Cheever, M.C., Greenberg, P.D. and Fefer, A. Potential for specific cancer therapy with immune T lymphocytes. J. Biol. Resp. Modif. 3:113-127, 1984.

33. In vivo effects of interleukin-2: BRMP Symposium. J. Biol. Resp. Modif. 3:455-527, 1984.

34. Mathé G., Amiel, J.L., Schwarzenberg, L., et al. Active immuno-therapy for acute lymphoblastic leukemia. Lancet 1:697-699, 1969.

35. Ellouz, F., Adam, A., Ciorbarn, F. and Lederer, E. Minimal structural requirements for the adjuvant activity of bacterial peptidoglycan derivatives. Biochem. Biophys. Res. Commun. 9:1317-1324, 1974.

36. Vosika, G.J. Clinical immunotherapy trials of bacterial components derived from Mycobacteria and Nocardia. J. Biol..Resp. Modif. 2:321-342, 1983.

37. Ribi, E. Beneficial modification of the endotoxin molecule. J. Biol. Resp. Modif. 3:1-9, 1984.

38. Oldham, R.K. and Smalley, R.V. Immunotherapy: The old and the new. J. Biol. Resp. Modif. 2:1-37

39. Terry, W.D. and Rosenberg, S.A., Eds. Immunotherapy of human cancer. Elsevier North Holland, New York, 1982.

40. Katano, M. and Torisu, M. New approach to management of malignant ascities with a streptococcal preparation OK-432. II. Intraperito-neal inflammatory cell-mediated tumor cell destruction. Surgery 93:365-373, 1983.

41. Micksche, M., Kokoschka, E.M., Luger, T., et al. Experimental and clinical studies with OK-432: A streptococcal preparation with immunomodulating properties. In: Human Cancer Immunology (Eds. B. Serrou), Elsevier North Holland, New York, 1982, pp. 31-54.

42. Bomford, R. and Moreno, C. Critical overview of the potential of various microbial polysaccharides for cancer immunotherapy. In: Augmenting Agents in Cancer Therapy (Eds. E.M. Hersh, M. Chirigos, M. Mastrangelo), Raven Press, New York, 1981, pp. 91-99.

43. Proctor, J.W., Auclair, B.G., Stokowski, L., Mansell, P.W.A. Comparison of the anti-tumor effects of glucan, BCG, and Levamisole. In: Immune Modulation and Control of Neoplasia by Adjuvant Therapy (Eds. M.A. Chirigos), Raven Press, New York, 1978, pp. 221-232.

44. Schultz, R.M., Papamatheakis, J.D., Chirigos, M.A. Tumoricidal effect in vitro of peritoneal macrophages from mice treated with glucan. In: Immune Modulation and Control of Neoplasia by Adjuvant Therapy (Ed. M.A. Chirigos), Raven Press, New York, 1978, pp. 241-248.

45. Aoki, T., Miyakoshi, H., Horikawa, Y. and Usuda, Y. Staphage lysate and lentinan as immunomodulators and/or immunopotentiators in clinical and experimental systems. In: Augmenting Agents in Cancer Therapy (Eds. E.M. Hersh, M.A. Chirigos and M. Mastrangelo), Raven Press, New York, 1981, pp. 101-112.

46. Oldham, R.K. Biologicals and biological response modifiers: The design of clinical trials. J. Biol. Resp. Modif. 4(2), 1985, in press.

47. Umezawa, H. Screening of small cell molecular microbial products modulating immune responses and bestatin. Recent Results Cancer Res. 75:115-125, 1980.

48. Umezawa, H. Small Molecular Immunomodifiers of Microbial Origin: Fundamental and Clinical Studies of Bestatin. Pergamon Press, New York, 1984.

49. Serrou, B., Cupissol, D., Flad, H., et al. Phase I evaluation of bestatin in patients bearing advanced solid tumors. In: Immunotherapy of Human Cancer (Eds. W.A. Terry and S. Rosenberg), Elsevier/North Holland, New York, 1982, pp. 453-458.

50. Ishihara, K. and Ikeda, S. Immunochemotherapy with bsetatin for squamous cell carcinoma and malignant melanoma. Proc. 13th International Cancer Congress, Vienna, 1983.

51. Kumamoto, Y. and Tsukamoto, T. Research on prevention of recurrence of superficial bladder cancer following TUR surgery: Efficacy of combined use of bestatin with bleomycin intravesical instillation. Proc. 13th International Cancer Congress, Vienna, 1983.

52. Ota, K. Randomized control clinical studies of bestatin treatment in leukemia. Proc. 13th Interntional Cancer Congress, Vienna, 1983.

53. Hersh, E.M., Chirigos, M.A. and Mastrangelo, M.J. Augmenting Agents in Cancer Therapy. Raven Press, New York, 1981.

54. Schroit, A.J., Hart, I.R., Madson, J. and Fidler, I.J. Selective delivery of drugs encapsulated in liposomes: Natural targeting to macrophages involved in various disease states. J. Biol. Resp. Modif. 2:97-100, 1983.

55. Fidler, I.J., Sone, S., Fogler, W.E., Smith, D., Braun, D.G., Tarcsay, L., Gisler, R.H. and Schroit, A.J. Efficacy of liposomes containing a lipophilic muramyl dipeptide derivative for activating the tumoricidal properties of alveolar macrophages in vivo. J. Biol. Resp. Modif. 1:43-55, 1982.

56. Deodhar, S.D., Barna, B.P., Ediger, M. and Chiang, T. Inhibition of lung metastases by liposomal immunotherapy in a murine fibrosarcoma model. J. Biol. Resp. Modif. 1:27-34, 1982.